CHER HAMPTON

The Somatic Therapy Toolbox

Your 28-Day Somatic Exercises Plan to Master the Mind-Body Connection for Effortless Relief from Trauma, Stress, Anxiety, and Chronic Pain in Just Minutes a Day

Disclaimer Notice:

Please note the information contained within this document is for educational and entertainment purposes only. All effort has been executed to present accurate, up to date, reliable, complete information. No warranties of any kind are declared or implied. Readers acknowledge that the author is not engaged in the rendering of legal, financial, medical or professional advice. The content within this book has been derived from various sources. Please consult a licensed professional before attempting any techniques outlined in this book.

By reading this document, the reader agrees that under no circumstances is the author responsible for any losses, direct or indirect, that are incurred as a result of the use of the information contained within this document, including, but not limited to, errors, omissions, or inaccuracies.

First edition

This book was professionally typeset on Reedsy.
Find out more at reedsy.com

Contents

BONUS: Your Free Gift

I'm only offering these bonuses for FREE to my readers. This is my way of saying thanks for your purchase. In these gifts, you will find valuable tools to BOOST your inner journey.

In the bonus section at the end of this book, you can find the link to download these bonuses for FREE.

#1 The Somatic Therapy Toolbox Audiobook

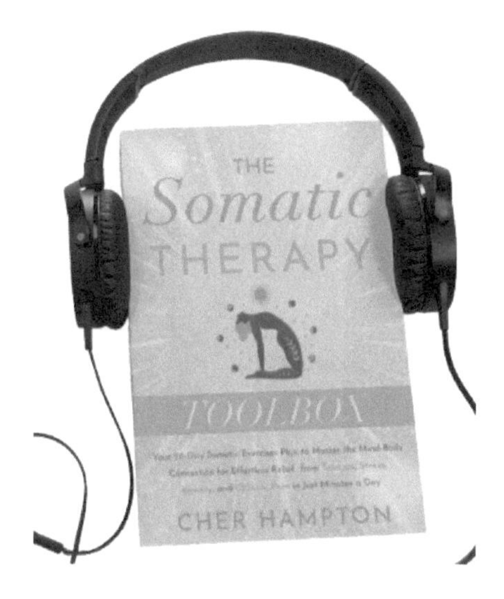

The Audio Version of This Book

#2 Nurturing Self-Care Guide

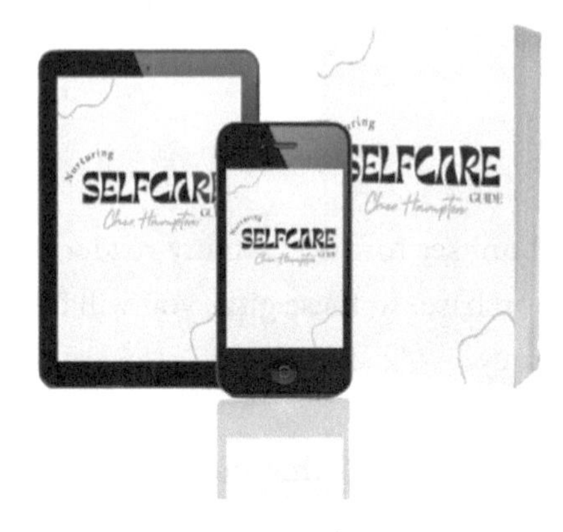

A Workbook with Special Meditations, Yoga Poses, and My Secret Self-Care Lists.

#3 Personality Development E-Course

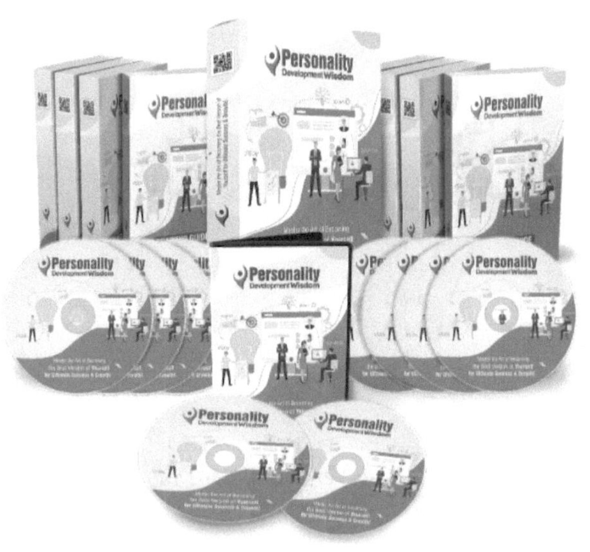

Master the Art of Becoming the Best Version of Yourself for Ultimate Success and Growth!

Introduction

Our bodies aren't just instruments through which we experience life but rather something that deserves to be explored, educated, and enriched. Our lives and experiences are inexorably linked to the physical sensations, movements, and rhythms that define our existence. As we explore the whole concept of somatic awareness, we begin to unravel the interconnectedness of our internal landscapes, laying the groundwork for profound self-discovery and growth.

The stresses and traumas we encounter in life can profoundly impact our physical and emotional well-being. Unresolved tensions and difficult experiences can literally become encoded into our musculature, breath patterns, and nervous systems. Over time, these imprints can manifest as chronic pain, anxiety, disconnection from our bodies, and a diminished sense of vitality. When we bring compassionate awareness to our somatic experience, we create space to process and release these accumulated stresses and traumas.

Anxiety is also increasingly prevalent. The constant barrage of stimuli and the weight of our fears and worries can leave us in a perpetual state of overwhelm. Somatic practices offer pathways to calm our overactive nervous system and digest the every day tensions we accumulate. Through conscious breathwork, gentle movement, and embodied meditations, we can activate our innate capacity to reset our equilibrium and reclaim our sense of grounded presence. This is a journey that we've treaded deeply into in our first two books, dedicating every page to fostering a richer understanding of the body-mind connection. Now, with this third installment, we continue building upon that rich foundation, further expanding our collective toolbox with an array of exercises, reflections, and insights.

The somatic practices in this workbook are not meant to be passively absorbed but actively explored and participated in. Every exercise has been carefully crafted to be experiential and interactive, guiding you through embodied inquiries, meditations, gentle movements, and reflective journaling. You'll be prompted to slow down, tune inward, and engage all of your bodily senses in the process of self-discovery.

This book's unique 28-day structure takes you on a step-by-step somatic journey designed to build your skills steadily and embodied awareness. Each day includes a new practice along with explanations, insights, and prompts to immerse yourself fully. By fully committing to and immersing yourself in this 28-day process, you can expect to reap profound, life-changing benefits. You will learn to destress and work through lingering traumas by befriending your body's innate healing capacities.

I'd like to emphasize that while some exercises may appear similar at first glance, they subtly differ from one another. This intentional design offers a versatile approach, allowing exploration of various facets of the mind-body connection. Repetition of thought processes in different ways can aid in fostering profound understanding and integration. So, don't be surprised if you encounter familiar elements—it's all part of the journey toward deeper self-awareness and promoting inner peace and well-being.

My hope for you is that by following this book, you can expect to gain a deeper sense of embodiment, be relieved of the tensions and stress that you've been carrying, awaken a stronger connection to yourself, and unlock the potential for growth and self-awareness, one somatic exercise at a time.

Understanding Somatic Therapy

"Life is always better in your body. Get out of your head."

— LEBO GRAND

The body has wisdom we will never fully comprehend. It holds memories, emotions, and the capacity for healing in ways that often elude the conscious mind. Somatic therapy, with its profound recognition of this body wisdom, offers a path to healing that is both ancient and urgently relevant today. As we delve deeper into "Understanding Somatic Therapy" in this third installment, our journey expands into the complex dance between the body and mind, revealing how the principles of neurological plasticity are not just scientific phenomena but also deeply intertwined with the healing processes facilitated by somatic therapy.

Neurological plasticity, or neuroplasticity, is the brain's remarkable ability to reorganize itself by forming new neural connections throughout life. Neuroplasticity is the brain's ability to change and adapt over time. It can be linked to the term "fire together, wire together," which refers to how connections between neurons become stronger when they are activated together repeatedly. So, when you learn to ride a bike, certain neurons in your brain are firing together as you practice this new skill. The more you practice, the stronger the connections become between those neurons that are firing together. It's like creating a new "wire" or pathway in your brain for riding a bike. The more those neurons fire together during practice, the more they wire together into an efficient neural network for that skill.

Neuroplasticity allows the brain to rewire itself and form new neural connections based on repeated experiences and learning. The firing together of neurons leads to the wiring together of those neural pathways, allowing the brain to physically change and adapt.

Somatic therapy leverages this intrinsic potential of our nervous system, guiding us through embodied experiences that reshape our brain's pathways, building resilience, and facilitating recovery from trauma, stress, and anxiety.

Somatic therapy is also a key contributor in healing trauma, stress, complex PTSD, and anxiety by acknowledging the profound wisdom of the body. It recognizes that our physical selves hold memories, emotions, and an innate capacity for healing that often eludes the conscious mind. When we embody practices such as mindful movement, breathwork, and sensory awareness, somatic therapy helps dissolve the barriers erected by traumatic experiences, anxiety, and chronic stress. Facilitating a reconnection with the sensations, emotions, and memories stored within our bodily tissues, this approach not only alters our mental landscapes but also literally rewires our brains, embodying the principles of neuroplasticity in deeply personal and transformative ways.

At its core, somatic therapy is an invitation to return to the body's innate intelligence, to listen deeply to its whispers and cries. It teaches us that our bodies are not mere vessels for our brains but integral partners in our emotional and psychological well-being. Mindful movement, breathwork, and sensory awareness help to dissolve the barriers erected by trauma, anxiety, and stress, allowing us to reconnect with the sensations, emotions, and memories that have been stored within our bodily tissues. This process of reconnection does not just alter our mental landscapes; it literally rewires our brains, thus reinforcing the principles of neuroplasticity in the most personal and transformative ways.

We must recognize that it offers more than just a method for personal growth. It provides a holistic framework for understanding the connection between the mind and body, illuminating how our thoughts, feelings, and physical sensations are inextricably linked. This recognition of the mind-body connection is crucial in approaching healing as a multidimensional journey that honors the complexity of the human experience. When we build that intimate and deeper connection with our physical selves, we become empowered to cultivate greater self-compassion, resilience, and a profound sense of inner peace. The practice of tuning into our body's signals teaches us to navigate life's challenges with grace and flexibility, embodying the very essence of neuroplasticity by adapting and thriving in the face of adversity.

The emphasis on bodily awareness and mindfulness paves the way for a more compassionate and attuned relationship with ourselves and our overall well-being. It is the very thing that helps us unlock new pathways to healing, resilience, and a more harmonious relationship with ourselves and the world around us. In this way, we can acknowledge that somatic therapy is not just a tool for healing; it is a testament to the incredible adaptability and potential that exists within each of us, waiting to be awakened.

Preparing For the Journey

"The partner of head is heart. Body has no opposite. In body, heart and head are one."

— GEORGI JOHNSON

I think you are brave for being here, for wanting to do the work, and for wanting to be a better you. It takes courage to want to work toward change. As you prepare for the 28-day journey ahead, remember that you are not alone in this process.

There's a lot of work that lies ahead, but it's nothing you can't handle. You will be challenged in the most remarkable of ways, but welcome all of it. Trust in yourself and the process, knowing that each step you take is a step toward a more fulfilling and authentic life.

To prepare for the journey ahead, start by setting clear intentions for what you hope to achieve during these 28 days. Reflect on what areas of your life you would like to focus on, whether it be physical health, emotional well-being, relationships, or personal development. Write down your goals and aspirations, and keep them somewhere visible as a daily reminder of what you are working toward. Here are some journal prompts to work through to help you set realistic goals for the journey ahead:

- What are your reasons for wanting to develop a greater mind-body connection? Is it to reduce stress, manage pain, increase energy, or something else?

- Think about a time when you felt really grounded and at ease in your body. What did that feel like physically?

- Do you tend to hold tension or stress in a particular area of your body (e.g., shoulders, jaw, stomach)? Getting curious about these holding patterns can help release them.

- What small daily habits or practices could you start incorporating to be more present and embodied (e.g., deep breaths, gentle stretches)?

- From head to toe, how do you feel? Are there any areas of tightness, discomfort, or ease? Meet whatever you notice with friendliness.

- What activities, movements, or environments help you feel more energized and alive in your body? How can you do more of those?

- If you strengthen your mind-body connection, what difference might that make in your life and well-being?

Starting small and avoiding judgment are key in beginning this somatic journey. As you begin this journey, create a supportive environment for yourself. Surround yourself with positivity and inspiration. Clear out any physical clutter in your living space that may be weighing you down. Make room for activities and practices that nourish your body, mind, and soul. Consider establishing a daily routine that includes time for exercise, meditation, journaling, or any other practices that help you feel grounded and centered. Here are some tips:

- **Start by identifying the things that might make it harder for you to try and stick to this new routine that you are trying to create.** For example, it might be harder for you to wake up early in the mornings, or you might feel too tired in the afternoons to follow through with the practice.

- **Find ways to combat these challenges.** Instead of waking up earlier each day, you'll find a way to squeeze the exercises into your afternoon; that way, you know you will show up wholeheartedly and consistently.

- **Determine how much time you're going to need.** If you decide that you are going to do your exercises in the morning, then you'll naturally need to wake up earlier than you usually do, so you will need to establish how much earlier you need to wake up.

- **Test out the new routine.** When doing this, you're going to need to remind yourself that you don't have to do everything all at once. start gradually, and as you get the hang of things, then you can start incorporating more. Also, don't be afraid to change things up. You'll realize that you no longer want to do things the way you thought you wanted to do them. That's okay; it's normal for routines to evolve and change with time.

Be as tender as you can with yourself throughout all of this. Change takes time, effort, and patience. There may be moments of doubt, resistance, or setbacks along the way, and that's okay. Feel what you are feeling without judgment. Embrace the journey as a learning experience, knowing that each challenge you face is an opportunity for growth and self-discovery.

Also, as you prepare for the 28-day journey ahead, be curious and open. Approach each day with a sense of wonder and possibility. Stay present in the moment, savoring the small victories and lessons that come your way. Trust in the process and in your inner wisdom to guide you toward a more empowered and authentic version of yourself.

Believe in your ability to transform your life and create the change you desire. You have everything you need within you to make this journey a success. Stay committed, stay focused, and, most importantly, stay true to yourself. The path ahead may be challenging, but with courage, determination, and self-compassion, you have the power to make this journey one of growth, healing, and transformation.

Notes on Consistency

Consistency is how you grow and how you keep at it. It's not enough to want something, be it healing, meeting a financial goal, or mastering the mind-body connection. You have to be willing to put in the work. The issue with most of us is that we are waiting for inspiration, for the perfect moment, while forgetting that circumstances or conditions will probably not always be ideal. We just have to have it within us to keep showing up, day after day, steadily bridging the gap between our minds and bodies.

Building consistency through a mind-body connection is about bringing awareness and harmony between your mental and physical states. Here's how it works:

The mind and body are intrinsically linked. Your thoughts influence your physical being, and your bodily sensations shape your mental state, but most of us live in a state of disconnect—we're stuck in the past, and the idea of "presence" is a foreign concept. Consistency in mind-body practices helps bridge this gap.

One approach is through meditation and mindfulness because it allows you to become aware of your thoughts as well as physical sensations like breathing. This heightened awareness allows you to notice when your mind is ruminating or when your body is tense and brings your attention back to the here and now. With consistent practice, you train yourself to be more present.

Physical practices like yoga, tai chi, or simple stretching also unite the mind and body. As you move and hold postures, you have to consciously guide your body while staying attuned to how you feel physically and mentally. The measured movements, linked to the breath, induce a state of mindfulness. Consistently doing these practices reinforces body awareness.

When your mind-body connection deepens through consistency, you develop greater self-knowledge and self-mastery. You can more easily recognize and work through emotional and physical tensions before they escalate. You respond to situations with poise instead of knee-jerk reactions. Ultimately, this coherence cultivates resilience, focus, and the ability to take wise action aligned with your values.

The mind-body link is a positive cycle—the more consistently you practice, the more integrated your mental and physical selves become. I want to highlight as well that we will never truly feel ready for the things that we want to do or the things that we have to do. The most important thing, however, is to just start. Start now, even if you're scared or uncertain. Start imperfectly. You don't have to have a pretty space or all of those other things that we tend to think we need to start. New things become less scary, less crippling, or less daunting when they aren't so new anymore. You've got this, and I believe in you!

Notes

Week 1: Establishing Awareness

"When we are grounded in our awareness, we can be more present with what we are experiencing in our bodies — in all the spaces that live between our head and our feet."

— RAEGAN ROBINSON

The small, seemingly mundane moments of our days are an opportunity for us to connect. This basically means that you can use moments through time to allow yourself to start noticing how your body responds to emotions and experiences and strengthen your inner resources to communicate that you are safe, balanced, and stable.

During your daily tasks, notice if you are present or spacing out. Gently bring your awareness back. What is in front of you? Notice the subtleties of what you are doing.

When you feel activated, notice it. What does this activation feel like in your body? Push your feet into the ground, slow down your breathing, and notice what that does to your physical sensations.

When you are rushing, take note of that. Lean into the backside of your body and toy around with the idea of letting everything in you slow down. How does that feel?

If you get too lost in your phone or a screen, catch yourself and then look at your surroundings. Look at one point in the room that you're in, or just look up at the sky.

These are the kind of moments called "low stakes." They are somewhat neutral, with less of an emotional charge. They can be more accessible for you to explore because there's less of an attachment to them. They allow you to start to notice how you automatically respond to life and gently invite more attention to your life experiences.

This is what makes you more resilient and because these are everyday moments, it gives you the chance to practice more consistently, strengthening your awareness each and every time so that you are able to come back to your body and yourself.

Day 1: Body Scan Meditation

A good benchmark for this exercise would be 15–20 minutes. It's ideal and sufficient to allow yourself to flow through the process without rushing yourself.

1. Close your eyes so that you can focus a little more, or if you prefer, you can lower or half close your eyes.

2. Bring awareness to your body, by inhaling and exhaling. Notice touch and pressure when your breaths make contact with your body. Be thorough in investigating each part of your body, taking as much time as you need.

3. When you're ready, take it as slowly as you want, intentionally breathe in. Move the attention to whatever body part you want to investigate and focus on. Whatever you choose to focus on, allow yourself to enjoy the process.

4. Some sensations that might appear include buzzing, tingling, or pressure. If you feel neutral, that's okay too. There are no right or wrong answers. Just tune in to what is present as best as you can without any judgment; all judgment does is put a different spin on things.

5. The main point is to be curious and open to whatever it is that you're noticing and then make space for yourself to intentionally release the focus of attention.

6. You might wander or drift off at times. It's great that you're noticing this, but don't judge yourself too harshly; just focus on redirecting your attention back to your body again.

7. When you're done, direct your attention to feeling your entire body breathing freely.

8. Open your eyes and allow yourself to move mindfully in this moment.

Questions to Reflect On

- *What did you notice about your body during the awareness exercise?*
- *How did you feel before and after the exercise?*
- *Did you notice any sensations or feelings that you weren't aware of before?*
- *How did it feel to intentionally focus on your body and its sensations?*
- *Did you find it challenging to stay focused on your body, and if so, how did you handle that challenge?*
- *How can you incorporate this practice of body awareness into your daily life?*

Day 2: Breath and Awareness

From the moment we are in our mother's wombs, there's an expanding and condensing rhythm that is tied together by moments of pause. These moments are the pulse of our universe; our breaths are an interior movement. At birth, when we draw that first gulp of air, we become one with the air around us; we inhale, and then we exhale that part that has become us into the world.

When we are much younger, we breathe with a remarkable kind of freedom, a kind of ease that just appreciates everything. This ease and freedom represent our innocence, but as we grow older, we lose some of that innocence because of the challenges that we sometimes find ourselves battling. We shut down and the first thing that is affected is the rhythm of our breath.

This disconnect from our breath indicates an unconscious attempt to control circumstances that are beyond our control. Thus, we go through our days with shallow breathing, suffocating, and sighing deeply just to recover. Or we may be so unconscious of our figure that we chronically contract our bellies, causing the breathing to tighten up in our chest.

When we teach ourselves to practice staying with our experiences with our breath and opening to each new sensation, whether it's pleasant or unpleasant, we automatically make ourselves more resources to encounter the difficulties that come our way. Breathing is about awareness, and awareness is about learning to breathe—learning to breathe through the confusion, the mess, the guilt, the joy, the bliss, and the agony of it all. In the following guided breathing exercise, we learn to take control and be more aware of our breathing.

Breathing Awareness Exercise

1. To begin the breathwork exercise, find a comfortable seated position with your chest and heart open and your shoulders resting softly on your sides. You can choose to close your eyes or lower your gaze, allowing your face and mouth to relax. Take a moment to notice where your attention is currently focused, acknowledging it without judgment, before gently and firmly turning your attention to the sensation of breathing.

2. As you breathe in and out, feel the body expand and contract without trying to control the breath in any way. Pay attention to where the breath is most vivid. Is it in the nostrils, chest, or abdomen? Rest there for a while.

3. It's normal for your mind to drift off to thoughts of the past or the future. When you notice this happening, let it all be and continue breathing. Each inward breath is an opportunity to begin again, and each outward breath is an opportunity to let go.

4. If your focus shifts to sensations in the body or other distractions, simply acknowledge what has captured your attention and gently bring your focus back to the breath. Let the breath be your anchor; feel the sensation of each breath as it moves in and through the body, and be with your life, one breath at a time.

5. Remember, this practice is about being present with your breath and not about controlling it. By bringing your attention to the breath and returning to it whenever your mind wanders, you can cultivate a sense of calm and clarity, helping you to be more present and focused in your daily life.

Reflection Questions

- *What is the most significant thing you noticed about your breath during this practice?*
- *Did you maintain your focus on your breath, or did your mind wander slightly?*
- *How did you feel before and after this practice?*
- *Did you experience any physical sensations or emotions during this practice?*
- *How can you use the sense of calm and clarity you cultivated during this practice to be more present and focused in your daily life?*

Day 3: Grounding Techniques

Grounding is focused on distraction strategies that help to reorient you to the here and now, helping you get through life's most stressful situations and get control over your most challenging emotions. Here are some techniques you can try:

- **Box breathing:** With this, you breathe in for four seconds, hold for four seconds, then breathe out for another four, hold again for four seconds, and repeat.
- **Moving:** You do a couple of exercises or stretches. For example, you can try jumping up and down, clenching and releasing your fists, walking slowly, and stretching different muscle groups one by one.
- **Carrying a grounding object:** This can be a small object like a rock, clay, a ring, a piece of cloth, or yarn. This is an item you touch or hold onto when you feel triggered.

- **Touch objects around you:** Notice the colors, weight, and temperature of materials. Compare the objects you touch. Which one is colder or warmer? Which one feels lighter?

- **Practice joyful focus:** Describe the steps of an action that you particularly enjoy doing, like making your favorite dish. Go through the step-by-step process as if you are giving someone else instructions on how to do it.

A Grounding Exercise: Doing Something You Enjoy

This breath-focused anchoring will help you feel steadied by the grounding rhythm of your inhalations and exhalations. You can use this whenever you need to regain your center and resolutely anchor into the present moment's stillness and stability.

1. Begin by finding a comfortable position, either seated or standing, and take a few deep breaths in and out to center yourself.

2. Close your eyes and bring to mind an action that you particularly enjoy doing. This could be anything, like making your favorite meal, going for a walk in nature, or playing a sport that you love.

3. Once you have your action in mind, start to visualize the steps involved in the process. For example, if you choose to make your favorite meal, start by visualizing the ingredients you'll need, the utensils you'll use, and the order in which you'll prepare each step.

4. As you visualize each step, pay attention to the sensations in your body. Notice any tension, discomfort, or relaxation that you feel as you imagine each step of the process.

5. Take your time with each step, allowing yourself to fully immerse in the

experience. If you get distracted or your mind starts to wander, simply bring your attention back to the present moment and continue with the exercise.

6. Once you've gone through all the steps of your chosen action, take a few deep breaths and come back to the present moment. Notice how you feel in your body and mind. Do you feel more grounded, centered, and present?

7. Finally, take a moment to reflect on the experience and how you can use this grounding exercise in your daily life. Whenever you feel stressed, anxious, or overwhelmed, you can use this exercise to bring yourself back to the present moment and cultivate a sense of calm and clarity.

Anchoring Yourself: An Exercise

1. Sit cross-legged and allow your spine to grow tall while feeling rooted and supported by the surface beneath you.

2. Close your eyes and bring your attention to your natural breathing rhythm. Don't try to change or control it; simply observe the flow of air moving in and out.

3. As you inhale, imagine drawing your breath down into your belly, allowing it to fully expand and rise like a balloon inflating.

4. With each exhale, feel your belly gently deflate and release, softening your body more deeply into a state of calm presence.

5. Continue breathing this way, visualizing your inhalations as anchors dropping into the depths of your belly, weighted and grounding.

6. You can enhance this by placing one hand on your belly to feel the rise

and fall as you slowly breathe in and out.

7. If your mind wanders, simply return your focus to the sensation of your anchoring breath moving through your body.

8. For several minutes, anchor into this gentle rhythmic flow, allowing the breath to balance and center your energy.

9. You can internally repeat a mantra like "In, anchor. Out, release," or simply the word "Anchored" on each exhale.

10. When you're ready, slowly open your eyes, carrying this anchored breath awareness into the rest of your experience.

Reflection Questions

- *How do you feel after taking a few moments to ground yourself and be present in the moment?*
- *Did you notice any physical or emotional sensations throughout the exercise?*
- *How might you incorporate this grounding exercise into your daily routine to help manage stress and anxiety?*
- *Did you find it challenging to stay focused on the visualization exercise? If so, are there any strategies you can use to help you stay present in the moment?*
- *What other mindfulness practices or self-care activities could you incorporate into your daily routine to support your overall well-being?*

Day 4: Progressive Muscle Relaxation

Progressive muscle relaxation (PMR) is used to reduce stress and promote relaxation by systematically tensing and then relaxing different muscle groups in the body. The goal of PMR is to help you become more aware of the difference between tension and relaxation in your muscles.

During a PMR session, you typically start by focusing on one muscle group at a time, such as your hands or arms. You tense these muscles tightly for a few seconds, then release the tension and let the muscles relax completely. This process is repeated for various muscle groups throughout the body, gradually moving from one area to another.

As you practice PMR regularly, you can develop a greater sense of bodily awareness and learn to release muscle tension more effectively. This can help reduce physical symptoms of stress, such as muscle tightness and pain, and promote a sense of overall relaxation and well-being.

Here is a step-by-step guided practice of PMR for you to follow:

1. Get a quiet environment. Take a few deep breaths to center yourself and relax.

2. Start by focusing on your hands. Clench your fists tightly, feeling the tension in your hands and forearms. Hold for a few seconds, then release and let your hands relax completely.

3. Move your focus to your biceps and upper arms. Tighten these muscles by flexing your arms, feeling the tension in your muscles. Hold for a few seconds, then release and let your arms relax.

4. Now, bring your attention to your shoulders. Shrug your shoulders up toward your ears, feeling the tension in your shoulder muscles. Hold

for a few seconds, then release and let your shoulders drop down.

5. Move up to your facial muscles. Scrunch up your face tightly, tensing your forehead, eyes, cheeks, and jaw. Hold for a few seconds, then release and let your face relax.

6. Continue with your chest, abdomen, back, thighs, calves, and feet, tensing each muscle group for a few seconds before releasing and relaxing.

7. Once you have gone through all the major muscle groups, take a few moments to focus on your entire body, noticing the difference between tension and relaxation.

8. Take a few deep breaths and enjoy the feeling of relaxation spreading throughout your body. Stay in this relaxed state for a few more minutes before slowly returning to your usual activities.

Reflection Questions

- *Which muscles do you hold tension in?*

- *How does your body feel after practicing PMR?*

Day 5: Sensory Awareness

Our senses are the very things that allow us to experience the lives that we are living. they are what allow us to be present, taste, see, feel, and savor the marvelous world around us. Sensory awareness plays a vital role in anchoring us in the present moment. When we focus on our senses, like feeling the ground beneath our feet, listening to the sounds around us, or observing the sights and smells in our environment, we become more attuned to the present moment.

When we move our attention to our senses, we naturally shift our awareness away from the distractions of the past or worries about the future. This heightened sensory awareness allows us to fully immerse ourselves in the richness of our immediate experience. It can help to ground us, reduce stress, and increase our overall sense of well-being.

Guided Practice of Tuning In

I want you to picture yourself in a serene, natural setting. Let's think of a peaceful forest clearing. Close your eyes and take a deep breath. Let's begin tuning into your five senses:

1. **Sight**: Slowly open your eyes and take in your surroundings. Notice the vibrant colors, the interplay of light and shadow, and the intricate details of nature around you. Allow yourself to truly see and appreciate the beauty that surrounds you.

2. **Sound**: Listen closely to the sounds of nature. Hear the rustling of leaves, the gentle chirping of birds, or the distant flow of a stream. Tune into each sound, letting them fill your senses and create a melody of tranquility.

3. **Touch**: Reach out and touch the elements around you. Feel the rough texture of tree bark, the softness of moss under your fingertips, or the cool breeze brushing against your skin. Explore different sensations and allow yourself to be fully immersed in the tactile experience.

4. **Smell**: Inhale deeply and savor the scents of nature. Notice the earthy aroma of damp soil, the sweet perfume of flowers, or the crisp freshness of the forest air. Let each scent awaken your senses and bring a sense of calm and grounding.

5. **Taste**: If you have a snack or drink with you, take a moment to indulge

your sense of taste. Notice the flavors, textures, and sensations as you eat or drink slowly. Pay attention to each bite or sip, savoring the experience fully.

Reflection Questions:

- *How did tuning into your senses enhance your experience of the present moment in this exercise?*
- *Did focusing on your senses help you feel more grounded or relaxed? In what ways?*
- *How can sensory awareness practices be incorporated into your daily life to cultivate mindfulness and presence?*

Day 6: Journaling Prompts for Body Awareness

Did you know that journaling is a great way to deepen the awareness and the connection that you have with your body?

Journaling is a powerful tool for deepening body awareness and helping us to tune into our physical sensations, emotions, and patterns that may otherwise go unnoticed. This practice offers a dedicated space and time to reflect on one's bodily experiences, fostering a deeper connection between the mind and body. The writing helps to slow down thoughts and feelings, making it easier to observe them more clearly.

Journaling serves as a bridge between the conscious and unconscious realms of our experience. It allows for an exploration of the body's subtle signals, which are often overshadowed by the busyness of daily life. Through journaling, one can begin to recognize patterns in physical sensations and emotional responses, offering insights into how the body holds and processes experiences. This awareness can be transformative, enabling individuals to identify stressors or triggers and to make more informed choices about their health and well-being.

Journaling also promotes mindfulness, a state of active, open attention to the present moment. When applied to body awareness, mindfulness through journaling encourages an attitude of curiosity and nonjudgment, allowing individuals to explore their physical and emotional landscape without criticism. This approach can lead to a more compassionate relationship with oneself, fostering a sense of acceptance and kindness toward your body.

Exercise: Journaling Prompts for Body Awareness

This exercise is designed to help you reflect on your physical sensations, emotions, and patterns in your body. Set aside some quiet, uninterrupted time for this practice, and approach it with an open heart and mind.

Physical Sensations

- Breathe for a couple of seconds. Notice any areas of tension or relaxation in your body without trying to change anything.

- Prompt: *What physical sensations am I experiencing right now? Where in my body do I feel them most intensely? Are these sensations familiar or new?*

Emotional Connection

- Reflect on any emotions you are currently feeling. Remember that emotions can also manifest physically in the body.

- Prompt: *What am I experiencing physically, and where in my body do I feel it? How do these emotions influence my physical sensations?*

Patterns and Triggers

- Consider if there are any recurring patterns in your physical or emotional responses. Think about what might trigger these patterns.

- Prompt: *Are there any patterns in how my body reacts to certain situations or emotions? What triggers these patterns, and how do they serve me?*

Responses and Coping Strategies

- Reflect on how you typically respond to the sensations and emotions you've identified. Consider if your coping strategies are effective or if there might be healthier alternatives.

- Prompt: *How do I usually respond to these physical sensations and emotions? Are there other ways I could respond that might be more beneficial for my well-being?*

Gratitude and Acknowledgment

- Finally, take a moment to express gratitude toward your body for all it does for you.

- Prompt: *What am I grateful for about my body today? How can I show my body appreciation and care?*

Day 7: Reflection and Integration

Reflecting on your experiences throughout your practice is what is going to allow you to integrate and make more sense of your experiences. You have to take the time to reflect and integrate what you've learned, as it will help you to move forward and make progress in your somatic therapy journey.

As you begin your reflection, try to focus on what stood out to you the most during the week. Maybe you had a breakthrough moment during one of the exercises, or perhaps you noticed a pattern emerging in your thoughts or behaviors. Whatever it is, take a moment to acknowledge it and give it the attention it deserves.

Once you've identified what stood out to you, try to explore it further. Ask yourself questions like the following: *What did I learn from this experience? How can I apply this knowledge to my life outside of therapy? What emotions came up for me during this experience, and why?*

It's normal to feel vulnerable and emotional during this process, so take breaks as needed and practice self-care. Remember that this workbook is just one part of your somatic therapy journey and that there is no right or wrong way to do it.

Finally, as you set your intention for the coming week, try to keep in mind what you've learned and how you want to apply it moving forward. Maybe you want to focus on cultivating self-compassion, or maybe you want to work on being more consistent in showing up for the practice. Whatever it is, make sure your intention is specific, measurable, and achievable. Here's what you can do:

Step 1: Reflect on the mind-body lessons and concepts that resonated most with you from what you've learned so far. Was it the importance of presence? The unity of mental and physical states? The value of consistent practice? Identify 1-2 key ideas you want to prioritize.

Step 2: Consider how you can apply those ideas to your own life in a practical way over the next week. Get specific about what actions or habits you can implement.

Step 3: Frame your intention as a specific, measurable statement. For example: *My intention is to meditate for 10 minutes every morning to build mental-physical presence* or *I will practice yoga three times this week to reinforce mind-body awareness.*

Step 4: Make sure your intention is realistic and achievable given your current circumstances. Start small if needed and build consistency over time.

Step 5: Write down your intention and put it somewhere you'll see it daily as a reminder.

Step 6: Schedule dedicated time slots in your calendar to uphold your intention through actual practice sessions. Treat these like important appointments.

Step 7: As you move through the week, periodically check in with your intention. Celebrate small wins, and don't beat yourself up over lapses—just refocus and reconnect with your purpose.

The key is to turn your intention into a concrete action plan with structured implementation. Remember, somatic therapy is a process, and progress happens one step at a time.

Notes

Week 2: Releasing Tension and Stress

"We have a brain in our belly, a very sophisticated one, and it responds to everything that's happened in our lives, so it accumulates a lot of stories over time."

— BONNIE BADENDOCH

We hold tension and stress everywhere in our bodies. It's in our hunched-up shoulders, our clenched jaw, and our tightened fists. Sometimes we don't even realize how much tension we are holding until we take a moment to pause and check in with our bodies.

Tension and stress can be caused by a variety of factors, including our daily routines, work, relationships, and even the news we consume. When we experience stress and tension, our bodies react by releasing stress hormones like cortisol and adrenaline. These hormones can be helpful in small doses, but when they are constantly being released, they can have negative effects on our physical and mental health.

In somatic therapy, we work to release tension and stress from our bodies so that we can feel more grounded and present in the moment. By doing so, we can reduce the amount of stress hormones our bodies are producing, which can help to improve our overall well-being. During this week, we will explore different techniques for releasing tension and stress from our bodies.

We will learn how to identify where we hold tension and stress, and we will practice techniques for releasing it. By the end of the week, you will have a better understanding of how to manage your stress and tension, and you will have a variety of tools to help you do so.

Day 8: Release and Shake Off

Shaking it off can be a powerful technique for releasing stress and tension from our bodies. When we shake our bodies, we activate our muscles and release built-up tension. This can help us to feel more grounded and present in the moment and can reduce the amount of stress hormones our bodies are producing.

Additionally, shaking it off can help us to let go of negative emotions and thoughts. When we shake our bodies, we allow ourselves to physically release the emotions and thoughts that are weighing us down. This can be a cathartic experience and can help us to feel more calm and centered.

So, whether you're dancing to Taylor Swift's "Shake It Off" or simply shaking your body out, know that you are taking an important step toward releasing stress and tension from your body. Give it a try and see how it makes you feel!

Release and Shake Off Exercise

1. Let's start by finding a comfortable and safe space where you can move freely without any distractions. Stand with your feet hip-width apart and your arms by your sides. Close your eyes and take a few deep breaths.

2. Begin shaking your hands and arms vigorously, shaking out any tension or stress you may be holding in your upper body. Allow your arms to flop around freely, and don't worry about how it looks or feels. Shake for about 30 seconds.

3. Next, shift your focus to your legs and feet. Begin shaking your legs from the hips down to your feet, allowing your knees to bend and your feet to stomp on the ground. Shake for about 30 seconds.

4. Now, move up to your hips and torso. Shake your hips and waist, allowing your spine to twist and your arms to swing around your body. Shake for about 30 seconds.

5. Finally, shake out your entire body all at once. Allow yourself to move freely and release any tension you may be holding in your body. Shake for about 1 minute.

6. Take a deep breath in and out, and notice how your body feels. Allow yourself to move around and stretch as needed. Remember that shaking it off can be a powerful technique for releasing stress and tension from our bodies, and it's okay to do this exercise whenever you need it.

Reflection Questions

- *How did your body feel before and after shaking it off?*
- *Did you notice any changes in your thoughts or emotions during or after the exercise?*
- *How can you incorporate this technique into your daily routine to help manage stress and tension?*

Day 9: Trauma and Tension Release Exercises

Trauma and tension release exercises (TREs) are used to help release tension, stress, and trauma stored in the body. These exercises involve movements that activate the body's natural tremor mechanism to release deep-seated tension and stress. The tremors are a natural and therapeutic way to release the accumulated tension in the body, and the exercises are designed to induce a sense of relaxation, calmness, and well-being. TRE can be a powerful tool for managing stress, anxiety, and trauma and can be incorporated into your daily routine to help you feel more centered and grounded. In short, TRE is a simple but effective way to release the tension and stress that accumulates in our bodies over time, providing a pathway to greater physical and emotional health.

Warning: While TRE exercises can be beneficial for many individuals, it's important to note that they may not be suitable for everyone. If you have any underlying medical conditions, physical injuries, or a history of trauma, it's recommended to consult with a qualified healthcare professional or a certified TRE practitioner before attempting these exercises on your own. They can provide guidance on whether TRE is appropriate for your specific situation and offer modifications or alternative approaches if necessary.

Shaking Free: A Trauma-Releasing Body Exercise

Preparation: Find a comfortable space where you can lie down on the floor. Have a mat, blanket, or towel available for padding. Ensure that you have enough space around you to allow for safe movement during the exercise.

Grounding (2–3 Minutes): Take a few deep breaths, focusing on the sensation of your body making contact with the floor. This will establish a sense of safety and grounding before starting the exercise.

Warm-up (5 Minutes): Engage in some gentle stretches or movements to prepare your body for the exercise. Pay particular attention to the areas around your hips, thighs, and lower back, as these will be the primary areas involved in the tremor response.

Activation Exercises (5–10 minutes): These exercises are designed to activate the tremor mechanism in the body. You should ideally spend 1–2 minutes on each exercise. Start with the following:

1. **Leg lift:** Lying on your back, extend one leg straight up toward the ceiling, keeping the other leg flat on the floor. Hold this position for five breaths, then switch legs. Repeat a few times.

2. **Pelvic tilt:** With both legs extended on the floor, gently tilt your pelvis upwards, creating an arch in your lower back. Hold for five to ten breaths, then release. Repeat it two times.

3. **Knee-to-chest:** Bring one knee toward your chest, keeping the other leg extended on the floor. Gently hug your knee toward your body, feeling the stretch in your lower back and glutes. Hold this for five to eight breaths, switch legs, and repeat it twice on each side.

Tremor Induction (10–15 minutes): After completing the activation exercises, return to lying flat on your back with your legs extended and arms at your sides. Take a few deep breaths and consciously relax your body, allowing any tension to release.

1. Focus on your breathing and scan your body for any areas that feel tense or contracted.

2. Gently engage your transverse abdominis (deep abdominal muscles) by gently pulling your navel toward your spine on the exhale. Don't forcefully suck in; just lightly engage these core muscles.

3. Allow your body to shake or tremble naturally without forcing the movement. The tremors may start small and gradually build in intensity.

4. Continue breathing deeply and surrendering to the tremors, letting

them move through without resistance for 10-15 minutes.

Integration (5 minutes): After the tremors have subsided, take a few moments to integrate the experience. Gently move your body, stretching any areas that feel tight or tense. Bring your awareness back to your breath and the sensation of your body on the floor.

When you feel ready, slowly come back to a seated position. Take a few deep breaths and allow yourself to transition back to your regular state of being.

A few safety tips to remember:

- Stop the exercise immediately if you experience any pain, discomfort, or overwhelming emotions.
- Stay hydrated and avoid practicing TRE on a full stomach.
- Proceed with caution if you have any injuries or physical limitations that may be exacerbated by the tremors.

Reflection Questions

- *How do you feel physically and mentally after practicing this exercise?*
- *Did you notice any particular areas of your body that were holding tension or stress?*
- *Will you incorporate this exercise into your daily routine to help manage stress and promote relaxation?*

Day 10: Self-Massage Techniques

Self-massage techniques can be an effective way to manage stress and promote relaxation. Massage helps to release muscle tension and increase blood flow throughout the body, which can help reduce stress levels and promote a sense of calm.

There are many different self-massage techniques that can be used to target specific areas of the body. For example, massaging the temples, neck, and shoulders can help relieve tension headaches and neck pain. Massaging the feet can help promote relaxation and improve sleep quality.

Incorporating self-massage into your daily routine can be a simple and effective way to manage stress. It can be done at home without the need for any special equipment or training. With regular practice, self-massage can become a valuable tool for promoting overall health and well-being.

Here is a step-by-step guide to a self-massage exercise that includes techniques for each of these areas:

Neck Massage

Neck Rolls

- Sit or stand comfortably with your back straight.
- Gently tilt your head to one side, bringing your ear toward your shoulder.
- Slowly roll your head in a circular motion, moving from one side to the other.
- Repeat this motion for 1–2 minutes, feeling the tension in your neck release.

Shoulder Squeezes

- Place your fingertips on your shoulders.
- Apply gentle pressure and begin to make small circular motions.
- Gradually increase the pressure as needed, focusing on tight or sore spots.
- Continue for 1–2 minutes, breathing deeply and relaxing into the massage.

Shoulder Massage

Shoulder Pinch

- Reach your right hand across your body to your left shoulder.
- Pinch the muscle between your fingers and thumb.
- Apply firm pressure and release, moving along the muscle.
- Repeat on the other shoulder, alternating sides for 1–2 minutes.

Shoulder Circles

- Place your fingertips on the tops of your shoulders.
- Slowly move your shoulders in circular motions, first forward and then backward.
- Focus on loosening any tightness or knots in the muscles.
- Continue for 1-2 minutes, adjusting the pressure as needed.

Foot Massage

Foot Roll

- Comfortably place a tennis ball or massage ball under your foot.
- Roll the ball from the base of your toes to your heel, applying gentle pressure.
- Focus on areas that feel tight or tender, pausing to massage them more deeply.
- Repeat on the other foot for 2-3 minutes.

Toe Stretch

- Sit and fatten your feet on the floor.
- Weave your fingers in between your toes and stretch them apart.
- Hold the stretch for a few seconds, then release.

- Repeat this stretch for each toe, focusing on flexibility and relaxation.

Reflection Questions

- *How does your body respond to self-massage?*
- *What emotions or sensations arise as you nurture yourself through touch?*

Day 11: Yoga For Stress Release

A yogi that I knew used to tell me that yoga is not just a physical practice, but a holistic approach to life. Yoga is a practice that has been around for thousands of years and is known for its ability to improve physical, mental, and emotional health. One of the most significant benefits of yoga is its ability to help us relieve and release stress that we are holding onto.

Stress can have a significant impact on our overall well-being. It can cause physical symptoms such as headaches, stomachaches, and muscle tension, as well as emotional symptoms such as anxiety, irritability, and depression. Yoga offers us a way to manage and reduce stress levels in a natural and holistic way.

Yoga is how we learn to quiet the mind and focus on the present moment. This helps us to become more aware of our thoughts and emotions and to develop a sense of calm and inner peace. The physical postures, or asanas, of yoga, also help to release tension and relieve physical symptoms of stress. It also incorporates breathing techniques, or pranayama, which can help to regulate our breath and calm the nervous system. This can have a profound effect on our overall sense of well-being and reduce feelings of anxiety and stress.

In addition to the physical and mental benefits of yoga, it is also something that allows us to communicate with a community of people. Practicing yoga with others can help us to feel supported and connected, which can be especially important during times of stress.

Flowing Our Way to Ease: A Yoga Sequence

With its physical postures, breathing techniques, and mental focus, yoga can help us find our way to renewed states of ease. Here is a yoga sequence you can try to help you with stress.

1. **Child's pose (balasana):** Begin on your hands and knees, with your knees apart and your big toes touching. Lower your hips back toward your heels and stretch your arms forward on the mat. Allow your forehead to rest on the mat, and take a few deep breaths.

2. **Cat/cow pose (marjaryasana/bitilasana):** From child's pose, come to a tabletop position on your hands and knees. As you inhale, arch your spine and lift your head and tailbone toward the sky (cow pose). As you exhale, round your spine and tuck your chin toward your chest (cat pose). Repeat for several rounds of breath.

3. **Downward-facing dog (adho mukha svanasana):** From tabletop position, lift your hips up and back to come into downward-facing dog. Spread your fingers wide and press into your palms and fingertips. Allow your head and neck to relax, and take several deep breaths.

4. **Standing forward fold (uttanasana):** From downward-facing dog, step your feet toward your hands and fold forward over your legs. Allow your head and neck to relax, and take several deep breaths.

5. **Mountain pose (tadasana):** From standing forward fold, slowly roll up to standing. Stand with your feet hip-width apart and your arms at your sides. Ground down through your feet and lift up through the crown of your head. Take several deep breaths.

6. **Tree pose (vrksasana):** From mountain pose, shift your weight onto your left foot and lift your right foot to rest on your inner left thigh. Press your foot and thigh together and bring your hands to your heart center. Take several deep breaths, then switch sides.

7. **Corpse pose (savasana):** Lie down on your back with your arms at your sides and your palms facing up. Allow your body to completely relax and release any tension. Stay here for several minutes, focusing on your breath.

Reflection Questions

- *How do I feel physically after completing this sequence? Do I notice any areas that feel more open or relaxed?*
- *How do I feel mentally and emotionally after completing this sequence? Do I feel more calm and centered?*
- *How can I incorporate these poses into my daily routine to support my physical and mental well-being?*

Day 12: Guided Imagery for Relaxation

I love to romanticize things. Some might even say that I am a little delusional. But in my defense, there's something magical about being able to escape our mundane reality and enter a world of our own creation. Guided imagery is one such tool that allows us to do just that. It's a powerful technique that involves the use of our imagination to create vivid mental images that can evoke a sense of calm and relaxation.

Whether it's picturing yourself lying on a beach with the sound of waves crashing in the background or visualizing yourself in a peaceful meadow surrounded by nature, guided imagery can transport you to a place where you feel safe, calm, and at ease.

In this session, we will explore the power of guided imagery and how it can help us relax and destress. We'll learn techniques to create our own mental images and use them to find peace and tranquility on an everyday basis.

A Visualization Exercise

1. You're going to need to find yourself a space where you'll be undisturbed for a while.

2. Take a few deep breaths, inhaling slowly through your nose and exhaling through your mouth. As you exhale, imagine all the tension and stress leaving your body.

3. Close your eyes and bring to mind a peaceful image. It could be a beach, a forest, a meadow, or any place that makes you feel calm and relaxed.

4. Visualize yourself in this place, using all your senses to make the image as vivid as possible. What do you see? What do you smell? What do you hear? What do you feel?

5. As you continue to visualize yourself in this peaceful setting, imagine a warm and soothing light entering your body. This light fills you with calmness, relaxation, and peace.

6. Focus on your breathing, taking slow and deep breaths. With each inhale, imagine the warm and soothing light spreading throughout your body, relaxing every muscle and releasing all tension.

7. As you exhale, imagine all negative thoughts and emotions leaving your body. Imagine them being carried away by the wind or washed away by

the waves.

8. Stay in this peaceful state for as long as you like, enjoying the sense of calm and relaxation that surrounds you.

9. When you're ready to end the exercise, take a few deep breaths and slowly open your eyes. Notice how you feel and appreciate the weightlessness and calm that you have created.

Reflection Questions

- *Did you find it easy or challenging to visualize yourself in a peaceful setting?*

- *Could you let go of negative thoughts and emotions throughout the exercise?*

- *What did you notice about your body and mind as you focused on your breathing?*

Day 13: Pilates for Tension and Stress Relief

Pilates is a low-impact form of exercise that helps you focus on building strength, flexibility, and mind-body awareness through controlled movements and breathing. Unlike yoga, which has origins in ancient Indian philosophy, Pilates was developed in the early 20th century by Joseph Pilates as a system of exercises to strengthen the body's "core" or deep abdominal muscles.

While both Pilates and yoga are centered around the idea of mindful movement and breathwork, there are some key differences:

- Yoga incorporates more static poses and stretches, while Pilates places more emphasis on flowing movements.
- Pilates exercises are often done on a mat or specialized equipment like

reformers, while yoga typically requires just a mat.
- The goal of yoga is more holistic well-being; Pilates is about physical conditioning.
- Yoga can have a spiritual component, whereas Pilates is more secularly focused on alignment and control.

Despite these differences, both of these practices can be very complementary for building somatic awareness and releasing tension.

Here is an easy Pilates exercise for you to do:

Gentle Spine Stretch

1. Lie on your back with your knees bent and feet flat on the floor. Arms can rest by your sides.

2. Inhale deeply through your nose, feeling your belly rise.

3. As you exhale slowly through pursed lips, begin curling your head and shoulders up off the mat while straightening your legs into a "V" position.

4. Inhale at the top of the stretch, opening across your upper back.

5. Exhale and slowly roll back down, vertebra by vertebra, drawing your knees back into your chest.

6. Repeat for 5–10 breaths, moving with control and focusing on lengthening the spine.

It seems deceptively simple, but it will do wonders in helping you release tension along your entire spine through flexion and extension. Go slowly, and only stretch as far as is comfortable for your body. The conscious breathwork will bring in that added element of awareness and release.

Day 14: Reflecting on Your Progress

You might feel a little different or you might even feel like you have made little to no progress at all, but either way, you made it through Week 2! Congratulations on taking this important step toward your well-being. As we progress through these somatic exercises, it is natural to wonder whether we are making any progress or not. Remember that it's all about consistency and it will take time to see results.

Simply take a moment to think about how you felt at the beginning of Week 1 and compare it to how you feel now. Did you notice any changes in your mood, energy level, or overall well-being? Maybe you noticed that you were able to focus better at work or that you are no longer holding tension in certain parts of your body

Even if you didn't notice any significant changes, remember that every moment and minute you dedicate toward your somatic practice counts toward your progress. Simply showing up for your practice, even when it feels difficult or unproductive, is an accomplishment in itself. So, give yourself a high five because I think that you're doing a pretty good job! But before we head off to the next week, I want you to properly set some intentions for yourself. Here are some questions that can guide you through the process

- What aspects of your life are causing you the most stress or tension currently?

- How can you incorporate practices like deep breathing, mindfulness, or other relaxation techniques into your daily routine to build resilience?

- Are there any specific situations or triggers that tend to deplete your resilience? How can you better prepare for or respond to those situations?

- What activities or hobbies can you engage in to help you recharge and replenish your mental and emotional reserves?

- Who in your support system can you rely on or reach out to when you're feeling overwhelmed or drained?

- What are some positive affirmations or mantras you can use to cultivate a more resilient mindset?

- How can you prioritize self-care practices like getting enough sleep, eating a balanced diet, and engaging in physical activity to enhance your overall resilience?

Notes

Week 3: Building Resilience

"Life doesn't get easier or more forgiving, we get stronger and more resilient."

— Steve Maraboli

You know, there's an old Japanese folk story that has stuck with me about resilience. It goes like this: When times get brutal, and it feels like everything is being stripped away, remember the mighty trees. Each year, they weather insane loss as their vibrant leaves get torn off by wind and cold, but those trees don't get bitter or buckle. Nope, they just stand their ground, staying rooted while patiently waiting for spring's inevitable rebirth. That's the resilience we all need to cultivate, friends. When crisis hits and the harsh elements threaten to break us down to bare branches, we've got to go tree-like: Shed what needs releasing, for sure, but keep anchoring deeper into our own grit and faith that rebirth and wholeness will return, no matter how wintery things get. It's a humble stubbornness that says, *I'll be stripped bare but never uprooted.*

Day 15: Resourcing Practice

Resourcing is a powerful practice that can help us feel empowered and better prepared to handle difficult life transitions. When we go through challenging times, it's easy to feel overwhelmed and powerless. We may feel like our whole world is falling apart, and we don't know how to cope with the situation.

Resourcing can help us develop a sense of inner strength and resilience, which can be incredibly helpful during times of stress and uncertainty.

The key to resourcing is learning how to access our inner resources. These resources might include our strengths, our values, our past successes, or our supportive relationships. By tapping into these inner resources, we can feel more grounded, more centered, and more capable of handling whatever life throws our way.

The biggest benefit of this practice is it allows us to plan for the inevitable messiness of life. We cannot control the particulars of every life stressor or every interruption that we encounter, but what we can do is plan for these challenges in advance so that we can weather these storms with greater ease and grace.

Resource Anchor: A Guided Practice

This following exercise involves you identifying a specific positive memory or experience that makes you feel strong and empowered and then using that memory as an anchor to ground yourself during times of stress.

1. Start with a few deep breaths, and then close your eyes. Think back to a time in your life when you felt really strong and capable. It could be a time when you accomplished something meaningful, overcame a difficult challenge, or felt deeply connected to someone you love.

2. As you recall this memory, try to engage all of your senses. What did you see, hear, smell, taste, and feel in that moment? Try to bring all of these sensory details to mind as vividly as possible. As you do so, imagine that you are stepping back into that moment and that you are experiencing all of those positive feelings once again.

3. Next, imagine that you are holding onto that memory as if it were an

anchor, grounding you and providing you with a source of strength and stability. Take a few deep breaths, and as you exhale, imagine that you are sinking deeper into that feeling of strength and resilience.

Whenever you feel stressed or overwhelmed in the future, you can use this resource anchor to help you feel more grounded and centered. Simply take a few deep breaths and then recall that positive memory, bringing all of those sensory details to mind once again. As you do so, allow yourself to sink deeper into that feeling of strength and resilience, knowing that you have the inner resources to handle whatever life throws your way.

Reflection Questions

- *How did recalling the positive memory make you feel?*
- *How do you think you can integrate this resource anchor into your daily life?*
- *What can you do to make sure you remember to use this resource anchor when you need it the most?*

Day 16: Emotional Regulation

When we feel triggered, instead of lashing out or shutting down, what we can teach ourselves to do is develop the skill of realizing that we have been triggered. When we recognize that we have been triggered, we can begin to take steps toward managing our feelings in a healthier way. This is where emotional regulation comes in, and it is a crucial part of our somatic practice. Learning how to regulate our emotions can help us navigate difficult situations with greater ease and can lead to improved relationships, increased self-awareness, and a greater sense of overall well-being.

An Exercise for When You're Carrying Heavy Emotions

Here is a step-by-step exercise that can help you regulate yourself when you are carrying heavy emotions:

1. Find a quiet, comfortable space where you won't be disturbed.

2. Close your eyes and take a few deep breaths, filling your lungs completely with air and releasing slowly.

3. Focus on the physical sensations in your body, starting with your feet and working your way up to your head. Notice any areas of tightness or discomfort and make a mental note of them.

4. Bring to mind the emotion you are experiencing and allow yourself to fully feel it without judgment. Acknowledge the feeling without trying to change it.

5. Visualize the emotion as a physical sensation in your body. Is it a heavy weight in your chest? A knot in your stomach? Allow yourself to fully experience this sensation.

6. Begin to regulate your breath, taking slow, deep breaths in through your nose and out through your mouth.

7. As you exhale, imagine releasing the emotion from your body with each breath. Visualize the sensation dissipating and leaving your body.

8. Continue this process of slow, regulated breathing until you feel a sense of calm and clarity.

9. When you are ready, slowly open your eyes and take a moment to ground yourself in the present moment.

Self-Soothing Breath Exercise

This simple breathing exercise can help calm your mind and body whenever you're feeling anxious, stressed, or overwhelmed:

1. Find a comfortable seated position, keeping your back straight but relaxed. You can sit on a chair, cushion, or cross-legged on the floor.

2. Bring your awareness to your breath. Notice the natural rhythm of your inhales and exhales without trying to change it.

3. Place one hand on your belly and the other on your chest. Breathe deeply so that your belly rises on the inhale and falls on the exhale.

4. As you inhale, count slowly to four. 1...2...3...4.

5. Then, exhale fully to a count of six. 1...2...3...4...5...6.

6. Continue breathing this way, inhaling for four counts and exhaling for six counts. Let your exhales be longer than your inhales.

7. If your mind wanders, gently bring your focus back to counting your breaths.

8. With each exhale, imagine releasing any tension, stress, or worries. Picture them leaving your body.

9. Keep your breathing smooth, steady, and relaxed throughout the exercise for 5–10 minutes.

10. End by taking one more full, clearing breath. Notice how you feel after this soothing breathwork.

This type of extended exhalation helps activate the parasympathetic nervous system, which controls resting, digesting, and relaxation responses. It's a simple but effective way to quickly self-soothe when you need it most.

Reflection Questions

- *How do you typically respond to strong emotions?*

- *Which of these strategies resonates with you for regulating emotions in a healthy way?*

- *What specific strategies or techniques can you implement when you start to feel triggered or overwhelmed by strong emotions? Make a list of at least 3-5 go-to strategies that you can refer to in those moments.*

Some examples could include:

- *deep breathing exercises*
- *going for a walk or engaging in physical activity*
- *journaling or writing down your thoughts and feelings*
- *calling a friend or loved one for support*
- *listening to calming music*
- *meditating on positive affirmations or mantras*
- *engaging in a hobby or activity you enjoy*

Day 17: Building Body Awareness Through Movement

Are you in your body? And when I say, "in your body," I don't just mean physically present or going through the motions of daily life. I'm talking about a deeper level of awareness, a profound connection to the sensations, movements, and rhythms of your body that often go unnoticed in the hustle and bustle of our busy lives.

Building body awareness through mindful movement is about tuning in to the language of your body, listening to its whispers and shouts, and honoring its wisdom. It's about cultivating a relationship with yourself that transcends the superficial and touches the core of your being. When we move mindfully, we invite ourselves to be fully present in each moment, to savor the sensations that arise, and to appreciate the intricate dance of muscles, bones, and breath that sustains us.

Body awareness is not just about knowing where your body is in space or how it looks in the mirror. It's about feeling the subtle shifts in tension and relaxation, noticing the ebb and flow of energy, and recognizing the messages that your body sends you through discomfort, pleasure, or pain. It's a practice of embodiment, of inhabiting your physical form with curiosity, compassion, and respect.

Are you ready to move with awareness, to dance with your breath, and to listen deeply to the language of your body? Here is a guided practice that is going to help you achieve that.

Pilates Core Flow

Pilates core flow is a form of exercise that focuses on developing core strength, flexibility, balance, and good posture. It involves a series of controlled movements that primarily target the muscles of the abdomen, lower back, hips, and thighs, as well as the muscles of the arms and shoulders.

Here is a 10 to 15-minute Pilates flow that you can include in your practice:

1. Start by standing with your feet hip-width apart and your arms at your sides. Take a deep breath in and as you exhale, gently activate your core muscles by drawing your belly button toward your spine.

2. Inhale and raise your arms overhead, reaching toward the ceiling. As

you exhale, hinge forward at the hips and fold forward, reaching your hands toward the floor. Keep your spine long and your core engaged.

3. Inhale and walk your hands forward, coming into a plank position with your wrists directly under your shoulders. Keep your core engaged and your hips level with your shoulders.

4. Exhale and lower down to the ground, keeping your elbows close to your sides. Inhale and lift your chest off the ground, coming into a cobra pose. Exhale and lower back down.

5. Inhale and press back into a downward-facing dog pose, with your palms and feet firmly planted on the ground and your hips lifted up toward the ceiling. Hold for a few breaths, then exhale and step your feet forward toward your hands.

6. Inhale and roll up to standing, one vertebra at a time, with your arms reaching overhead. Exhale and lower your arms back down to your sides.

7. Repeat the flow 5-10 times, moving with your breath.

Tips:

- Remember to keep your core engaged throughout the flow to support your spine and protect your lower back.
- If you have any injuries or limitations, be sure to modify the exercises as needed or consult with a healthcare professional before starting the flow.
- Always listen to your body and move at a pace that feels comfortable and safe for you.

Reflection Questions

- *How does your body respond to mindful movement?*
- *What insights did you gain about your body's capabilities and limitations?*

Day 18: Cultivating Joy and Gratitude

Joy is not finite. It is not something that comes and goes with time but something that I believe is an inherent part of who we are. Joy for the sake of joy is what I believe in and strive for every day. Cultivating joy and gratitude changes our entire outlook on life. When we embrace these states of being, we invite positivity, contentment, and peace into our daily experiences.

Gratitude allows us to appreciate the small moments, the simple pleasures, and the beauty that surrounds us. It shifts our focus from everything that we think we don't have to what is abundant in our lives. Joy as well is like a beacon of light that brightens even the darkest of days. It is contagious, spreading warmth and happiness to those around us. When we cultivate joy, we open ourselves up to something lovely in our lives. We begin to notice the tiny sparks of delight in the mundane, finding reasons to smile and laugh amidst the chaos.

Together, joy and gratitude are a dynamic duo. They remind us to celebrate the simple joys, express gratitude for the blessings, and find moments of levity in the midst of challenges.

Thank You to Life: A Gratitude Practice

When was the last time you let the words "thank you" fall from your lips, not out of obligation, but out of genuine appreciation for the beauty of life and the kindness of others? In this "thank you to life" practice, take a moment to reflect on the moments that have evoked gratitude within you.

Begin by finding a quiet space where you can sit comfortably. Close your eyes and take a few deep breaths, allowing yourself to ground in the present moment. Think back to a recent interaction or experience that touched your heart or brought a smile to your face.

Now, grab a pen. Start by writing down three things you are thankful for today. These can be big or small, personal or universal. Reflect on why each of these things fills you with gratitude and how they have impacted your day or your life in general.

1.

2.

3.

Next, shift your focus to the people in your life who have made a difference, no matter how small. Write a short thank-you note to someone who has supported you, inspired you, or simply been a positive presence in your life. Express your appreciation for their kindness, their wisdom, or their love in a few heartfelt sentences.

As you write these thank-you notes, let your heart guide your words. Feel the warmth and gratitude radiate from within you as you acknowledge the abundance of blessings that surround you. This practice of recognizing and expressing gratitude can deepen your connection to the beauty of life and amplify the joy and appreciation you feel each day.

Holding Space for Joy: An Exercise

Dear Joy, You're so welcome in this place of my heart, where your light can shine brightly, and your presence can be felt deeply. In this exercise, we will explore ways to expand your capacity for joy, inviting more of this precious emotion into your life and embracing it wholeheartedly.

We are going to start with connecting to the power of our breath, Take a few deep breaths to center yourself and focus on the present moment. As you inhale, envision yourself breathing in positivity, love, and light. As you exhale, release any tension or negativity that may be weighing you down.

Now, think about a recent moment that brought you pure joy. It could be a simple pleasure, a heartfelt connection, or a beautiful experience that made your soul sing. Close your eyes and relive that moment in your mind, savoring every detail and allowing the feelings of joy to wash over you.

Next, grab a pen. Write down three things that consistently bring joy into your life. These could be activities, people, places, or aspects of yourself that uplift your spirit and fill you with happiness. Reflect on why these sources of joy are meaningful to you and how you can invite more of them into your daily routine.

1.

2.

3.

Now, set an intention to seek out joy in unexpected places. Challenge yourself to find moments of delight and wonder in the mundane aspects of your day-to-day life. Notice the beauty in small details, the laughter in simple interactions, and the magic in ordinary moments.

P.S. When joy finds you and when you find it, I hope you intentionally hold on to it.

Reflection Questions

- *What are you grateful for in this moment?*

- *How does cultivating gratitude and joy contribute to your resilience?*

Day 19: Strengthening Your Nervous System

Our nervous systems are constantly communicating with us and asking us deeply important questions. They're asking us questions like:

- Am I safe?
- Do I feel safe enough to rest?
- Do I feel safe enough to play?
- Do I feel safe enough to surrender into the arms of love?
- Am I safe enough to be fully present in this moment, this body, and this breath that I am holding?

Our nervous systems heal in slowness and softness. It can take time and a whole lot of tenderness, but slowly, gradually, we can teach our nervous systems that it is safe to rest and safe to be in general.

High-Intensity Interval Training

High-intensity interval training (HIIT) is a form of cardiovascular exercise that involves short bursts of intense activity followed by periods of rest or low-intensity exercise. This type of exercise has been shown to increase the production of brain-derived neurotrophic factor (BDNF), which is a protein that supports the growth and survival of neurons in the brain and helps to improve cognitive function. Additionally, HIIT has been found to reduce inflammation in the body, which can contribute to nervous system dysfunction.

Now, let's move on to the 15-minute HIIT exercise.

Warm-up (3 minutes): Start with a light jog or jumping jacks to get your heart rate up and muscles warmed up.

High-intensity exercise (30 seconds): Choose an exercise that gets your heart pumping, such as sprinting, jumping squats, or burpees. Do the exercise as fast and as hard as you can for 30 seconds.

Rest (30 seconds): Take a break and catch your breath.

Low-intensity exercise (60 seconds): Do a low-intensity exercise, such as walking in place or doing lunges, for 60 seconds.

High-intensity exercise (30 seconds): Choose a different high-intensity exercise and do it for 30 seconds.

Rest (30 seconds): Take a break and catch your breath.

Low-intensity exercise (60 seconds): Do a different low-intensity exercise for 60 seconds.

Repeat steps 2-7 (5 times): Repeat the high-intensity, rest, and low-intensity exercises for a total of 5 rounds.

Cool-down (2 minutes): Finish with a slow walk or stretching to bring your heart rate down and prevent injury.

By doing this HIIT exercise, you are stimulating your nervous system and increasing the production of BDNF. This exercise can also help to reduce inflammation in the body, which can lead to a healthier nervous system overall. Stay hydrated and listen to your body. If you experience any pain or discomfort, stop the exercise.

HIIT is not going to be everyone's cup of tea, so there's a gentler exercise that you can try. You can opt for tapping exercises, also known as the Emotional Freedom Technique (EFT) or tapping therapy. It's about gently tapping specific points on the body while focusing on specific thoughts or emotions. Doing these movements will help you to activate and regulate the nervous system, reduce stress and anxiety, and promote relaxation.

Getting Started

Identify the issue, emotion, or physical sensation you want to address. Rate its intensity on a scale of 0 to 10, where 0 represents no intensity and 10 represents the highest intensity.

The Tapping Sequence

- **Karate chop point:** Start by tapping the fleshy part of your hand, just below the little finger, while repeating a simple setup statement out loud, such as "Even though I have this [issue/emotion/sensation], I deeply and completely accept myself."

- **Eyebrow point:** Using two or more fingertips, tap just above and to one side of the nose at the beginning of the eyebrow.

- **On the eye:** Tap on the bony ridge on the outside corner of the eye socket.

- **Under the eye:** Tap on the bony ridge under the eye, about 1 inch below your pupil.

- **Under the nose:** Tap on the area between the bottom of your nose and the top of your upper lip.

- **Chin point:** Tap on the crease area between the bottom of your lower lip and the top of your chin.

- **Collarbone point:** Tap just below the hard ridge of your collarbone, about 1 inch down and 1 inch over from the U-shaped notch at the top of your breastbone.
- **Under the arm:** Tap on the side of your body, about 4 inches below the armpit.
- **Repeat:** Repeat this sequence while focusing on the issue, emotion, or sensation you identified. You can modify the wording as needed, such as "This [issue/emotion/sensation] is starting to fade" or "I am releasing this [issue/emotion/sensation]."

After completing the sequence, take a deep breath and reassess the intensity of the issue, emotion, or sensation on the 0 to 10 scale. If the intensity has decreased, you can continue with additional rounds of tapping or move on to other techniques. The best part about these is that they are gentle and incredibly easy to learn, and you can do them anywhere.

Reflections

- *How does your body respond to practices aimed at supporting nervous system health?*
- *What sensations or shifts do you notice in your body and mind?*

Day 20: Expressive Art Therapy

Art therapy is a form of psychotherapy that involves creating art as a means of expressing yourself and exploring emotions and experiences. The focus is not on creating a masterpiece but rather on the experience of creating. It is a process-oriented therapy that values the journey of creating art more than the final product. The creation of art can be a powerful tool in therapy as it allows you to express your most intimate feelings and emotions in a nonverbal way. Focusing on the process of creating rather than the end product, art therapy offers you the opportunity to connect with yourself on a deeper level and to express your innermost thoughts and feelings.

Exercise: Art Therapy at Home

Materials Needed

- paper or canvas
- paints, markers, pencils, or any other art supplies you enjoy using
- a comfortable and quiet space to work in
- optional: music or other relaxing aids

Instructions

1. Set aside at least 30 minutes of uninterrupted time for this exercise.

2. Choose a color or art supply that resonates with you in the moment.

3. Begin creating whatever comes to mind. Paint something like a picture of a pretty flower, a house, or your favorite place. Don't worry about the end product or whether it looks "good" or not. Just focus on the process of creating.

4. As you work, notice any thoughts or feelings that arise. Allow yourself to express them through your artwork.

5. If you feel stuck or don't know where to begin, try starting with a simple shape or line and see where it takes you.

6. If you feel comfortable, you can also try experimenting with different art materials or colors to express different emotions.

7. Keep working until you feel ready to stop. You can also set a timer for a specific amount of time if that helps.

8. Take a step back and observe your creation. Notice any patterns, colors, or symbols that stand out to you.

9. Reflect on the experience. How did it feel to express yourself through art? Did any insights or realizations come up for you? Write them down if you like.

Remember, this exercise is about the process of creating rather than the end product. Don't judge yourself or your artwork. Simply allow yourself to explore and express.

Reflection Questions

- *Did you find the art therapy exercise helpful in expressing your thoughts and feelings? Why or why not?*

- *What patterns or symbols did you notice in your artwork? How do they relate to your current state of mind?*

- *What did you learn about yourself through this exercise? How can you apply this knowledge to your daily life?*

Day 21: Review and Adjustments

The one thing that you should always try to remember is that it is also completely okay if you feel that certain exercises don't resonate with you. We all have individual needs, and we are different in the sense that our bodies will respond differently to different things. So spend the rest of today looking through all of the exercises that you did this week and ask yourself these questions:

- What resilience-building techniques were most impactful for you this week?

- How will you adapt your self-care routine based on your experiences and observations?

- Were there any exercises that you found particularly challenging or uncomfortable? What made them difficult for you?

- Are there any exercises that you found particularly helpful or effective? Why do you think they worked well for you?

- Did you notice any patterns or themes in your responses to the exercises this week? What insights did you gain about yourself?

The goal of this toolbox is to help you find what works best for you and your unique needs. Keep experimenting with different techniques and approaches until you find what resonates with you. And above all, be kind and patient with yourself throughout the process.

Notes

Week 4: Integration and Mastery

"What happens when people open their hearts? They get better."

— HARUKI MURAKAMI

I like to believe that if I am present, I will be able to bear witness to the most spectacular moments of my life. The moments that make me realize in awe that life is actually good and that I am quite lucky that I get to be me. Being fully present can be challenging, especially when we are dealing with difficult emotions or experiences. However, it is in those moments of presence that we can begin to integrate and heal. This week, we will be cultivating awareness and creating space for integration and healing.

Day 22: Mindfulness and Meditation

I have heard a lot of things about meditation, ranging from the absurd to the most sensible and wisest things. It wasn't until I tried it for myself that I truly understood its power. Meditation is a practice that has been around for thousands of years, and while it can seem intimidating or overwhelming at first, it is actually quite simple. At its core, it is about cultivating a sense of presence and awareness. It is a way to connect with ourselves and the world around us on a deeper level. Today, we're going to explore various mindfulness and meditation exercises that can help you integrate these practices into your daily life. Remember, the goal is not to become an expert meditator overnight but to simply start where you are and allow the practice to unfold naturally.

Guided Mindful Meditation: An Exercise

You are here, in this body that carries you, in the breath you hold and release, in the present moment. Take a moment to settle into this space, allowing your body and mind to relax.

1. Begin by getting comfortable in your seated or lying down position. Adjust your posture so your spine is straight yet relaxed. Allow your hands to rest gently in your lap or at your sides.

2. Take a deep breath in through your nose, drawing air fully into your belly. Exhale slowly through pursed lips. With each exhale, imagine any stress or tension leaving your body.

3. Now, bring your attention fully to the sensations of breathing. Observe the gentle rise of your belly on the inhale and the relaxing fall on the exhale. Don't try to change your breath; simply tune into its natural flow.

4. As you breathe in, you may notice the subtle coolness of air entering your nostrils and the feeling of your lungs expanding. As you exhale, perceive the stream of warm air exiting your mouth or nose.

5. With each cycle of breath, you are here, anchored in the present moment experience of your body. You have nowhere to go, nothing to do, but simply be here and breathe.

6. If your mind wanders into thinking, gently escort your awareness back to the breath. Use the anchor of the inhale and the exhale to remain grounded. You don't have to follow or resist thoughts, simply let them arise and pass without clinging.

7. With every in breath, you are nourishing your body with life-giving oxygen. As you exhale, you are releasing any tensions, worries, or constrictions. Breathe in calm. Breathe out anything that no longer serves you.

8. For the next several minutes, continue this focused breathing practice. When you notice your mind has drifted, simply return to the next incoming breath. Use each inhalation to regather your attention and each exhalation to shed distractions.

9. You may become aware of sounds, physical sensations, or fleeting emotions. Simply notice them with an attitude of friendly curiosity, then return your concentration to the anchor of your breath.

10. Whenever you're ready, you can gently open your eyes or keep them closed for a few more breaths. Take one last deep, clearing breath and welcome yourself back into the present moment feeling calm, centered, and at peace.

Reflection Questions

- *What did you notice during the mindfulness meditation practice?*
- *How does mindfulness support your overall well-being and resilience?*

Day 23: Breathwork

I believe that we don't heal ourselves so that we are able to handle the bad days. I believe that we heal so that we are able to hold more space for joy, life, and the tiny bursts of wonder that exist in between. And that's where breathwork comes in. Our breath is intimately connected to our physical, emotional, and mental states. Manipulating these patterns allows us to access deeper states of consciousness and release emotional blockages that may have been holding us back.

Different breathing techniques have different effects. For example, rapid, shallow breathing from the chest tends to increase feelings of anxiety, stress, and tension in the body. In contrast, slow, deep belly breathing activates the relaxation response—lowering blood pressure and heart rate and producing a calming effect on the mind.

Other breathwork practices use a conscious circular breathing pattern to induce a mild hypoxic state in the body. This increased oxygen deprivation can lead to an altered state of consciousness, allowing the release of stored emotional traumas and limiting beliefs. Holotropic breathing follows this model of using faster, continuous inhales and exhales to enter a nonordinary state of awareness.

Other techniques like box breathing (inhale four counts, hold four, exhale four, hold four) and alternate nostril breathing help balance the left and right hemispheres of the brain. This can increase mental clarity, concentration, and equanimity. Yogic practices like breath retention build energetic capacity and presence.

Using these ancient breathwork modalities with intention, we start to find that we are able to access insights and truths that were previously hidden from view. We may experience a profound sense of release and catharsis as we breathe through old patterns, emotions, and stories we've been carrying.

Our breath is sacred; it is the bridge between our inner and outer experiences of life. When we learn to harness it skillfully, we open to living with more vibrancy, freedom, and delight.

A Breathwork Exercise

1. Find a quiet, comfortable place to sit or lie down where you won't be interrupted for at least 10–15 minutes.

2. Close your eyes and take a few deep breaths in through your nose and out through your mouth. Allow your body to relax and release any tension you may be holding.

3. Begin to breathe in and out through your nose, focusing on the sensation of the air moving through your nostrils.

4. As you continue to breathe, visualize a bright, warm light filling your body with each inhale. Imagine this light spreading through your entire body, from the top of your head to the tips of your toes.

5. With each exhale, visualize any negative thoughts, emotions, or energy leaving your body as dark smoke or clouds.

6. As you breathe, focus on the sound and rhythm of your breath. You can use a mantra or affirmation to help you stay centered and focused.

7. Continue this practice for 10–15 minutes, allowing yourself to fully relax and surrender to the experience.

8. When you're ready, slowly begin to bring your awareness back to your body and your surroundings.

9. Take a few deep breaths in and out, and when you're ready, open your eyes.

10. Take a moment to reflect on your experience and notice any shifts or changes in your body and mind.

Reflection Questions

- *How did your body and mind respond to the breathwork exercises?*
- *What emotions or sensations arose during the practice?*

Day 24: Energy Work and Healing Modalities

Your energy has far more power than you could ever imagine. Every thought, feeling, and vibration that we have out there contributes to our current reality.

Energy work is a holistic healing method that focuses on balancing the energy systems in the body to promote physical, emotional, and spiritual well-being. It is based on the premise that the human body is composed of several interconnected energy systems that function together to maintain health and vitality. These energy systems include the chakras, meridians, and aura. The chakras are the seven energy centers located along the spine that correspond to different physical and emotional aspects of our being. Each chakra is associated with a specific color, sound, and element, and when they are balanced, they promote health and vitality.

The meridians are the pathways through which energy flows in the body, and they are often used in acupuncture and acupressure to release blockages and restore balance.

The aura is the electromagnetic field that surrounds the body, and it reflects our physical, emotional, and spiritual state. Energy work practitioners use various techniques such as meditation, visualization, and breathwork to balance the energy systems in the body and promote healing.

Energy work is significant in holistic healing because it recognizes that our physical health is closely connected to our emotional and spiritual well-being. When our energy systems are balanced, we feel more grounded, centered, and connected to our higher self. This, in turn, promotes healing on all levels of our being, leading to a more vibrant and fulfilling life.

Guided Exercise to Identify and Release Energy Blockages

1. Sit or lie down, and take a few deep breaths, relaxing your body with each exhale.

2. As you breathe, focus on the area of your body where you feel the most tension or discomfort. This could be your neck, shoulders, lower back, or anywhere else.

3. Imagine that you are holding a ball of energy in your hands. This energy represents any negative emotions or blockages that you are holding onto in your body.

4. As you inhale, visualize the ball of energy moving from your hands into the area of your body where you feel tension or discomfort. Imagine the energy breaking up any blockages or tension in that area.

5. As you exhale, imagine the ball of energy leaving your body, taking with it any negative emotions or blockages that were released during the exercise.

6. Repeat this process for each area of your body where you feel tension or discomfort. Allow yourself to fully release any negative emotions or blockages that are stored in your body.

7. When you are finished, take a few deep breaths and slowly open your eyes. Take note of how you feel, both physically and emotionally. If you still feel out of place, it's okay, with time you'll get used to it and gradually it will become easier.

Visualization Techniques to Promote Energy Flow and Vitality

1. Lie down comfortably.

2. Close your eyes and take a few deep breaths, letting go of any tension or stress in your body.

3. Imagine a radiant, pulsating energy source at the center of your being, like a brilliant star or a glowing ember.

4. Visualize this energy source expanding and radiating outwards, filling every cell and fiber of your body with its warm, revitalizing essence.

5. Focus your awareness on your root chakra, located at the base of your spine. Picture a deep, earthy red color pulsating in this area, representing your connection to the Earth and your sense of grounding and security.

6. Move your attention to your sacral chakra, a few inches below your navel. Envision a vibrant orange swirl, symbolizing your creativity, passion, and sensuality.

7. Shift your focus to your solar plexus chakra in your upper abdomen. Visualize a golden yellow sun radiating confidence, willpower, and personal power.

8. Bring your awareness to your heart chakra at the center of your chest. See a verdant green energy, representing love, compassion, and your ability to nurture yourself and others.

9. Move to your throat chakra in your neck area. Picture a serene blue hue, symbolizing your ability to communicate effectively and express yourself authentically.

10. Concentrate on your third eye chakra located in the center of your forehead. Imagine a deep indigo color representing your intuition, wisdom, and spiritual insight.

11. Finally, focus on your crown chakra at the top of your head. Visualize a brilliant violet light, symbolizing your connection to the divine and your highest potential.

12. As you focus on each chakra, repeat a positive affirmation related to its qualities and functions. For example, for the heart chakra, you might repeat, "I am open to giving and receiving love."

13. Continue this process until you have visualized all of your chakras and feel balanced, energized, and in harmony with your inner self. Below is also a brief explanation of each of your chakras and what they mean.

Root chakra (Muladhara) is located at the base of the spine. Visualize a bright red spinning vortex of energy.

Sacral chakra (Svadhisthana) is a few inches below the navel. Picture a vibrant orange wheel spinning.

Solar plexus chakra (Manipura) is in the upper abdomen area. Think of a brilliant yellow disc radiating.

Heart chakra (Anahata) is at the heart center in the middle of the chest. See an emerald green vortex spinning with love.

Throat chakra (Vishuddha) is in the throat area. Try picturing a sky-blue spinning wheel representing communication.

Third eye chakra (Ajna) is in the center of the forehead. Visualize an indigo light representing intuition.

Crown chakra (Sahasrara) is at the top of the head. Picture a luminous violet or white vortex of divine connection.

As you focus on each chakra, repeat a positive affirmation related to that chakra. For example, for the heart chakra, you might repeat, "I am open to giving and receiving love.

Continue this process until you have visualized all of your chakras and feel balanced and energized.

Healing Modalities

Healing modalities are various techniques and practices that we can use to promote physical, emotional, and spiritual well-being. Let's look at some popular modalities and their principles:

Reiki: Reiki is a Japanese healing technique that uses the practitioner's hands to channel energy into the client's body. The energy is believed to promote healing by restoring balance and harmony to the body's energy centers. The principles of Reiki include promoting relaxation, reducing stress, and helping the body to heal itself.

Acupuncture: Acupuncture is a traditional Chinese medicine practice that involves inserting thin needles into specific points on the body. The needles are believed to stimulate the body's energy flow and promote healing. Acupuncture is used to treat a variety of physical and mental health conditions, including pain, anxiety, and depression.

Acupressure: Acupressure is similar to acupuncture in that it involves stimulating specific points on the body to promote healing. However, acupressure uses finger pressure instead of needles. It is often used to relieve pain, reduce stress, and promote relaxation.

Reflexology: Reflexology is a practice that involves applying pressure to specific points on the feet, hands, and ears. The theory behind reflexology is that these points are connected to different organs and systems in the body and that stimulating them can promote healing and balance. Reflexology is often used to reduce stress, improve circulation, and promote relaxation.

Each of these healing modalities has its own unique principles and techniques, but they all share a common goal of promoting health and well-being.

Self-Healing Exercise

Here is a simple self-healing exercise that you can practice for relaxation and rejuvenation:

1. Find a quiet and comfortable place where you can sit or lie down.

2. Close your eyes and take a few deep breaths, inhaling through your nose and exhaling through your mouth.

3. Visualize a bright light at the top of your head. This light represents positive energy and healing.

4. Take a deep breath and imagine the light flowing down through your body, starting at the top of your head and flowing down through your neck, shoulders, chest, abdomen, hips, legs, and feet.

5. As the light flows through your body, imagine it clearing away any negative or stagnant energy, leaving you feeling refreshed and rejuvenated.

6. Continue to breathe deeply and visualize the light flowing through your body for several minutes.

7. When you are ready, slowly open your eyes and take a few more deep breaths.

Another technique for clearing and replenishing your energy field is called grounding. Here's how to do it:

1. Find a quiet and comfortable place where you can stand on the ground with bare feet. Grass or soil is ideal, but if that's not possible, a wooden floor or carpet will also work.

2. Stand with your feet hip-width apart and your arms at your sides.

3. Close your eyes and take a few deep breaths.

4. Visualize roots growing out of the soles of your feet and extending deep into the earth.

5. Imagine that you are connected to the earth's energy and that it is flowing up through your feet and into your body, filling you with positive energy and vitality.

6. Stay in this position for several minutes, breathing deeply and feeling the energy flowing through your body.

7. When you are ready, slowly open your eyes and take a few more deep breaths.

These simple energy work exercises can be practiced regularly to promote relaxation, rejuvenation, and overall well-being.

Guided Energy Meditation

This is a guided energy meditation that is focused on helping you connect and channel healing. You're going to need a quiet space where you can allow yourself to be fully immersed in this practice. Close your eyes and take a few deep breaths, inhaling through your nose and exhaling through your mouth.

Visualize a bright light at the top of your head. This light represents positive energy and healing. Take a deep breath and imagine the light flowing down through your body, starting at the top of your head and flowing down through your neck, shoulders, chest, abdomen, hips, legs, and feet.

As the light flows through your body, imagine it clearing away any negative or stagnant energy, leaving you feeling refreshed and rejuvenated. Visualize this light as a healing force that is bringing peace and harmony to your entire being.

Now, let's focus on connecting with this healing energy. Visualize a beautiful, radiant light that surrounds you. This is the universal energy of healing and love. Feel it flowing through you, filling you with a sense of peace and calm.

As you breathe in, visualize this healing energy entering your body, flowing through your veins and arteries, and reaching every cell in your body. Imagine it filling you with health and vitality.

As you breathe out, release any negative thoughts or emotions. Let go of any stress, anxiety, or tension that you may be holding onto. Allow this healing energy to take its place, filling you with love and light.

Now, imagine that you are a channel for this healing energy. Visualize the light flowing through you and out into the world, touching the lives of others and bringing healing to all those who need it.

As you continue to breathe deeply, imagine this healing energy growing stronger and more vibrant with each passing moment. See it spreading out into the world, radiating peace and love to all those around you.

Stay in this position for as long as you like, breathing deeply and feeling the energy flowing through your body. When you are ready, slowly open your eyes and take a few more deep breaths.

Remember that you can practice this guided energy meditation regularly to promote relaxation, rejuvenation, and overall well-being. Thank you for joining me today.

Reflection Questions

- *How did I feel after practicing the guided energy meditation?*
- *Did I encounter any challenges today, and how did I handle them?*
- *What positive experiences or interactions did I have today, and how did they impact me?*

Day 25: Inner Child Work

Your inner child needs you.

They need you to advocate for your growth.

They need you to nurture the fears that reside within you.

They need you to provide a structure and a schedule.

They need you to pave space for healing and thriving in all aspects of your life.

They need you to allow yourself to be creative, fun, and imaginative.

They need you to believe in the best and most spectacular version of yourself.

They need you to surround yourself with an endless amount of support and love.

Inner child work is a process of reconnecting with and healing our childhood wounds. It is based on the idea that our childhood experiences shape who we are as adults because when we understand and address the unresolved emotional issues from our past, we can heal our inner child and move forward with a greater sense of well-being.

The inner child holds our memories, emotions, and experiences from childhood; the parts of us that feel vulnerable, scared, and emotional. Trauma and negative experiences can create wounds that we carry into adulthood and affect our ability to form healthy relationships and live fulfilling lives. Inner child work invites us to process, explore, and compassionately identify the negative beliefs and patterns that we have developed as a result of our childhood experiences and learn to reframe them in a positive light. This can involve confronting painful memories, acknowledging difficult emotions, and learning to release pent-up anger, sadness, and fear.

The process can be challenging, as it often involves confronting painful emotions and memories that have been buried for years, but the benefits are rich and plenty. This healing work allows us to be the kind of people who are intentional in boundary setting, the kind of people who have more fulfilling relationships, and live more authentically.

Writing Exercise: Exploring and Nurturing Your Inner Child

There is power in the pen. Sometimes, we don't have the language or the vocabulary to intimately explore those buried memories, to talk about how they made us feel or how they potentially impacted us. But when we sit in silence with pen and paper, it becomes a lot easier. Here is a writing exercise that we're going to do to explore and nurture our inner child.

Step 1: Connect with your inner child: Imagine yourself as a child, perhaps around the age of 5 or 6. What did you look like? What were your favorite things to do? What did you enjoy playing with? Try to visualize yourself as vividly as possible and imagine your inner child sitting in front of you.

Step 2: Write a letter to your inner child: Begin writing a letter to your inner child. Start by acknowledging how special and loved they are and how much they mean to you. Then, write about some of the positive experiences you had as a child, such as happy memories or moments when you felt loved and cared for. You may also want to share some of the dreams and aspirations you had as a child.

Step 3: Comfort and reassure your inner child: Next, write about some of the difficult experiences you had as a child. Perhaps there were times when you felt scared, lonely, or misunderstood. Write about these experiences with empathy and understanding, and reassure your inner child that they are not alone and that you are there for them.

Step 4: Nurture your inner child: Finally, write about ways that you can nurture and care for your inner child. This may involve engaging in activities that you enjoyed as a child, such as coloring, drawing, or playing games. You may also want to write about ways that you can practice self-care and self-compassion in your daily life, such as taking time for yourself or setting healthy boundaries.

Step 5: Be with your experience: After you have finished writing, take a few moments to reflect on your experience. How did it feel to connect with your inner child? Did any new insights or emotions come up for you? What can you do to continue nurturing your inner child in your daily life?

Reflection questions

- *What emotions or memories arise when connecting with your inner child?*

- *How can you offer support and healing to your inner child moving forward?*

P.S. If you would like to discover more about your inner child and heal her/him, you can best read one of my following books:

- **Healing Your Inner Child First:** Becoming the Best Version of Yourself by Letting Go of the Past, Overcoming Trauma, and Feeling Worthy
- **Inner Child Healing Workbook:** Your Companion Workbook with Exercises, Meditations, and Prompts to Let Go of the Past, Overcome Trauma, and Cultivate Self-Love

Day 26: Establishing Support Systems

When we surround ourselves with supportive people, we create a space where we can be our true selves without fear of judgment or rejection. This kind of environment can be a powerful force in our lives, giving us the courage to pursue our dreams, overcome challenges, and grow as individuals. It's also a place where we can find comfort and solace during difficult times, knowing that we have people who care about us and are there for us when we need them most.

Building a supportive environment isn't always easy, especially if we've been hurt or let down by people in the past. It can take time to find the right people and build those relationships, but the effort is well worth it. One way to start is by being intentional about the people we surround ourselves with. We can seek out individuals who share our values and interests and who uplift and inspire us. We can also work on being the kind of person we want to attract into our lives—someone who is kind, supportive, and compassionate.

Identifying Supportive Individuals

People who have people are the luckiest yet, would you not say? So, just take a moment to reflect on the people in your life who support you and uplift you.

- Who are the individuals who make you feel safe and loved?

- Who do you turn to when you need advice or a listening ear?

It's important to acknowledge the people who bring positivity into our lives and to express gratitude for their presence. Consider reaching out to them and letting them know how much they mean to you.

Communicating Needs and Boundaries

Your needs and boundaries will never be too much for someone who says that they care about you. That's because they aren't. It's important to communicate your needs and boundaries to others because it helps establish healthy relationships. By sharing what you're comfortable with and what you're not, you can create an environment of mutual respect and trust. It also helps prevent misunderstandings and conflict. When people know what you need and what you expect, they are better equipped to meet your needs and respect your boundaries. Here are some tips for communicating your needs and your boundaries:

- **Take time to reflect on your needs and boundaries beforehand so that you can clearly communicate them to others.**

- **Be assertive but not aggressive.** State your needs and boundaries with confidence and clarity, but also be willing to listen to the other person's perspective.

- **Be open to negotiation and compromise.** Recognize that others may have different needs and boundaries, and be willing to find a middle ground that works for both parties.

- **Remind yourself that boundary setting doesn't have to be static.** It's okay if they change and it's okay as well for you to adjust them as you go. You are only human, a person in progress, so it's only normal to find that what you once thought you wanted is not it.

Building Your Support Network

Making friends as an adult can be challenging, and building a support network can seem daunting. Some of you may not have good relationships with your families. In such instances, what can you do? After all, you cannot go through life alone. Even the best of people need help.

Look out for social activities that interest you, such as joining a club or community group. This can provide a great opportunity to meet like-minded people and start building connections.

Volunteering is also a great option; this can be a great way to meet new people while giving back to your community. Some other ideas include:

- attending networking events in your industry or profession
- joining a recreational sports league or fitness class
- attending a local meetup group for a hobby you enjoy
- taking a class or workshop on a subject that interests you
- attending social events hosted by your workplace or alumni group
- joining a book club or writing group
- attending concerts, festivals, or other community events
- joining online communities or forums related to your interests
- attending religious or spiritual gatherings in your community
- considering using a friend-finding app or website to connect with others looking to make new friends

I'm not saying it's going to happen overnight. But you're going to have to be persistent in your efforts. Just because it might not have worked out with some people doesn't mean you should give up altogether. You will find your tribe, your people, because they're somewhere out there waiting for you as well.

Creating Your Support Network

Creating a support plan can be a great way to ensure that you have a network of people who can help you during difficult times when you're feeling ill or need someone to pick up the kids from school when you can't make it. Here are some steps you can take to create a support plan that outlines specific ways in which support system members can assist you as you heal:

- **Identify your current group of people**: Start by identifying the people in your life who you can count on for support. This could include family members, friends, coworkers, or members of a support group.

- **Establish what your needs are**: Think about the specific ways in which you need support. Do you need someone to talk to when you're feeling anxious? Do you need help with practical tasks, such as running errands or cooking meals?

- **Communicate your needs**: Once you've identified your support system and determined your needs, communicate this information to your support system members. Let them know what they can do to help you, and be specific about your needs.

- **Set boundaries**: It's important to set boundaries with your support system members to ensure that they are providing the help you need without overwhelming you. Let them know what you're comfortable with and what you're not.

- **Adjust as you go**: Over time, your needs may change, and your support system may evolve. Review your support plan periodically to ensure that it still meets your needs, and don't be afraid to make adjustments as necessary.

Self-Advocacy and Empowerment

At the end of the day, it's all up to you to do the work and to fight as ferociously as you can to get to that emotionally healthy state. You need to advocate and empower yourself because if you don't, no one else is going to do it for you. You can do that through the power of the spoken word—affirmations. You can talk yourself into a state of empowerment, and these are some of the encouragements that you can start with:

- My inherent worth is unshakable, and I vow to honor myself through nurturing self-kindness and love.

- The healing journey is mine to navigate, and I'm taking the empowered reins to create the positive transformation I seek.

- Difficulties will arise, but I'm made of resilient stuff—overcoming obstacles is within my capabilities.

- I place deep trust in my inner wisdom to make self-honoring choices, and I will speak up for my needs.

- Wholeness, fulfillment, and radiant wellness are my birthright, and I'll steadily tend to cultivate that each new day.

- My commitment to growth means pausing to appreciate the incremental wins, letting each one fuel me forward.

- I acknowledge my progress and celebrate even the smallest victories along the way.

- I will continue to learn and grow, and I am committed to my healing journey.

- I choose to focus on the positive and stay hopeful, even in difficult times.

- I am capable of creating the life I want and deserve, and I will not give up on myself.

Day 27: Creating a Personalized Self-Care Plan

You owe it to yourself to be gentle toward and to be kind and intentional about what you choose to flow within and outside of you. You owe yourself at least 30 minutes in your day where it all gets to be about you and no one else, and yes, you don't even have to feel guilty about it. Creating a personalized self-care plan is a great way to prioritize your needs and make sure you're taking care of yourself in a way that works for you. You have at least five different types of self-care cups that you can fill and replenish. These cups include your spiritual, emotional, physical, mental, and intellectual needs. Here's a breakdown of how you can tend to each of these needs:

Spiritual Self-Care

This involves nurturing your inner self and finding deeper meaning in your life. Incorporating somatic practices can help you feel more grounded and centered. Here are some examples:

Spiritual Self-Care

- practicing mindful meditation or yoga to connect with your body and soul
- going for a walk in nature to feel more connected to the world around you
- journaling to reflect on your thoughts and feelings

Social Self-Care

This involves all the ways in which you nurture your relationships with others and build a supportive community. You tend to your social self-care cup by:

- attending a group fitness class or dance class to connect with others while moving your body
- practicing partner yoga or massage with a loved one to deepen your connection
- listening during conversations to stay present and connected with others

Emotional Self-Care:

You need healthy ways to relate to your emotions. Emotional self-care is how you learn to express yourself and learn to control your emotions so that they, in turn, don't end up controlling you. A lot of these ideas below are exercises you've done already in the workbook, so you can refer back to them if you need a refresher.

- practicing deep breathing or progressive muscle relaxation to calm your nervous system
- moving your body to release pent-up emotions, such as dancing or shaking
- using body-based visualization techniques to help you process difficult emotions

Physical Self-Care:

This self-care is all about honoring your body's need for nutrition and rest. You fill your physical self-care cup by:

- practicing yoga or stretching to improve your flexibility and mobility
- regularly exercising and finding ways to move in which you enjoy
- getting a massage or practicing self-massage to release tension and improve circulation

Mental/Intellectual Self-Care:

Learning new things can help us feel empowered. Incorporating somatic practices into your intellectual life can help you feel more present and focused, which can improve your cognitive function. Here are some ideas:

- practicing mindful breathing or body scanning to improve your focus and concentration

- engaging in creative activities, such as painting or writing, to stimulate your imagination
- practicing mindful movements, such as tai chi or qigong, to improve your mind-body connection and mental clarity

Creating Your Own Personalized Self-Care Routine

Self-care is something that should be individual to our own unique needs. So now what you can do is use the knowledge that you have of the various forms of self-care to create something that speaks to you on a personal level. I've gathered some prompts that are going to help you get started:

- What are some physical self-care practices that you enjoy? Will you have to go to a specific place away from your home?

- What are some emotional self-care practices that help you feel grounded and centered? How can you make them more special?

- What are some social self-care practices that help you connect with others and build relationships? How can you schedule these practices into your week?

- What are some spiritual self-care practices that help you feel more connected to yourself and the world around you? How can you integrate these practices into your daily life?

- What are some mental/intellectual self-care practices that help stimulate your mind and keep you engaged?

Once you have the answers to these questions, get yourself a planner and start mapping out the various activities into different days. You can, for example, dedicate a week to a specific form of self-care, or you can combine them, e.g., having a physical self-care day and an intellectual self-care day at the same time (you go for a foot massage and take your favorite book with you to read). It's all about flexibility and doing things that make your soul happy.

Reflection Questions

- *Do you feel any guilt about your self-care practices? What can you do to combat that?*

- *How much more creative can you get with your self-care?*

Day 28: Practicing Self Compassion

Self-compassion is that tender place that holds space for the parts of us that we have been taught to deny; it embraces them with love and drives the shame away from the steering wheel.

There is no better feeling than the feeling you experience when you finally learn to love all of those parts that you initially hated. To come back to yourself in a way that feels more deeply right than anything else. So many of us have encountered instances where we are shamed for being who we are or for experiencing what we experience, and that shame is what drives that disconnection from our core parts. it causes so much discomfort, so much fear and anxiety. It is what is at the root of our worst coping mechanisms and behaviors.

But when we take all of those and bring them into the light, we learn that all this shame that we are carrying was never ours to hold to begin with. The more familiar we become with the various parts of ourselves, the less control the external environment has over us.

You are in charge and get to drive the change. You get to walk toward the people, things, and experiences that can bring you healing and joy. You get to walk toward all the self-compassion you need.

Guided Self-Compassion Meditation

This is a guided meditation that you can do sitting on the floor, sitting on a chair, or even sitting on the couch. Once you have decided which place is going to be best for you to practice, I want you to breathe in and imagine inhaling calmness and peace. As you exhale, release any tension or negative thoughts that may be weighing you down. Feel the rhythm of your breath, the gentle rise and fall of your chest, grounding you in this moment.

Then you're going to bring your attention to your body. Notice any areas of tension or discomfort, and without judgment, send them soothing thoughts of kindness and compassion. Picture a warm, golden light surrounding those areas, soothing them with each breath you take.

Turn your attention toward your emotions. Acknowledge any feelings that arise within you —whether they are positive or negative. Hold space for them; welcome them with an open heart, knowing that it is okay to feel whatever you are feeling in this moment. Offer yourself words of comfort and understanding, like "I am here for you" and "You are not alone."

Picture a moment when you felt truly loved and cared for. It could be a memory of a friend's comforting hug, a kind word from a loved one, or a moment of self-compassion you have experienced before. Allow that feeling of warmth and acceptance to fill your heart, enveloping you in a cocoon of love.

As you bask in this feeling of love and compassion, repeat the following affirmations silently to yourself:

- "There is room for love and kindness here in this heart."
- "I forgive myself. I forgive myself. I. Forgive. Myself."
- "I am enough. Just as I am. Just where I am"
- "I lovingly hold myself to treat with gentleness and care."

Continue to breathe deeply and slowly, letting these affirmations sink into your being, nurturing your soul with each breath. Feel a sense of peace and acceptance wash over you, knowing that you are deserving of your own love and compassion.

When you are ready, gently bring your awareness back to the present moment. Wiggle your fingers and toes, gradually opening your eyes. Take a moment to thank yourself for taking this time to nurture your inner self with kindness and compassion.

Overcoming Barriers to Self-Compassion

Shame, unworthiness, a lack of self-forgiveness, and not feeling worthy enough are so often the things that prevent us from loving ourselves as we deserve to show and give ourselves. All of these barriers are the very things that keep us feeling small and insignificant in our own lives, but we can fight against them by practicing the following:

- **Hold space for forgiveness:** You can't keep beating yourself up about the things that happened in the past. You have to learn to forgive yourself so that you can move on. It's going to be hard, but the hard parts are what we need to get through to find our way to the easier bits.

- **Watch how you talk to yourself:** These things, like shame, thrive in toxicity; they want you to talk yourself down. They want you to keep moving like a shadow around yourself, not like you are the main character. So when you catch yourself about to say something negative to yourself, reframe it into something with positive undertones or something more neutral.

- **Learn to be with your experience:** Our capacity to be with life and life's experiences is congruent with our ability to come to a state of acceptance for what they were. Things happen, and life happens, but we can't keep ruminating. We can't keep wishing things were different. Let yourself feel angry, sad, and regretful, and when the time comes, let go and go on.

Small, baby steps, you certainly won't win the whole fight in one go. but as long as you are breathing to see another day, another sunrise, and another sunset, you will survive.

Reflection Questions

- *How do you typically relate to yourself during difficult times?*
- *How can you cultivate greater self-compassion and kindness toward yourself?*

Notes

Celebrating Progress and Continued Growth

"I can do this. "But what if you can't?" I ask myself. Then something strong inside of you will save you."

— CHER HAMPTON

A big part of learning how to be happy is about learning to be excited. Learn to be excited about both the big and small things: your coffee in the morning or a meet-up with a friend. Celebrate your daily wins, such as doing the things that you thought you couldn't do. Be in love with falling in love and fall in love with life. I hope that this book was something like that for you. I hope that the tools and practices you've learned feel like seeds planted in the fertile soil of your daily life—seeds that will bring forth joy and, yes, a whole lot of excitement for what lies ahead.

Somatic therapy is not just a set of techniques; it's a way of being and a constant conversation between mind and body that doesn't end on the last page of a book. It's about nurturing a lifelong relationship with yourself, filled with curiosity, compassion, and the joy of discovery.

So, as you conclude this 28-day program, you have to keep in mind that true growth and self-care are ongoing processes. They're not a one-stop shop. The insights and practices you have acquired should not be confined to these 28 days alone but should be integrated into your daily life. Commit to continuing with everything, nurturing the mind-body connection, and prioritizing self-care as an integral part of your journey.

Also, remember to celebrate your accomplishments. You should be your biggest cheerleader. The insights you gained and the growth you experienced are a testament to your dedication and commitment to personal growth. Each exercise, each moment of presence, and each lesson learned have contributed to your transformation and will continue to do so as you go through life. Reflect on the progress you have made, the awareness you have cultivated, and the newfound understanding of your somatic experiences.

As you continue to weave these practices into your life, I hope that your relationship with your body, your emotions, and the world around you begins to shift in subtle yet profound ways. I hope that you carry the excitement of all of this into each new day, finding delight in the unfolding of your own story, just as you would cherish the blooming of a flower you've tended from seeds.

And now, as you gently close the cover of this book and step forward, I invite you to think about the following questions:

1. What have been the most significant shifts in your body awareness since starting this 28-day somatic journey?
2. How have the practices in this toolbox helped you to connect with your present-moment experiences in a deeper way?
3. In what ways have you noticed your responses to stress or difficult emotions changing?
4. What were the moments that brought you unexpected joy or insight,

and how can you invite more of those moments into your life?

5. As you reflect on your path to falling in love with life, what are the small pleasures that you've started to appreciate more?

6. How can you continue to cultivate excitement for both the mundane and the magnificent aspects of your daily experiences?

7. What are the next steps you intend to take to further deepen your somatic practice and enrich your connection to yourself and the world around you?

May you find your guiding light. The place you go to remind yourself of the many "why's" behind why you choose to do all this healing work. Thank you for allowing me to be a part of your exploration of living. Keep nurturing your excitement for life because it is the heartbeat of joy and the essence of a life well-lived.

Notes

BONUS: Your Free Gift

I'm only offering these bonuses for FREE to my readers. This is my way of saying thanks for your purchase. In these gifts, you will find valuable tools to BOOST your inner journey.

#1 The Somatic Therapy Toolbox Audiobook

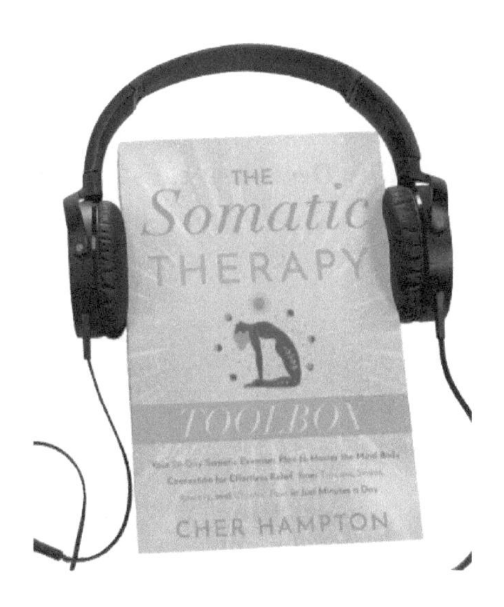

The Audio Version of This Book

#2 Nurturing Self-Care Guide

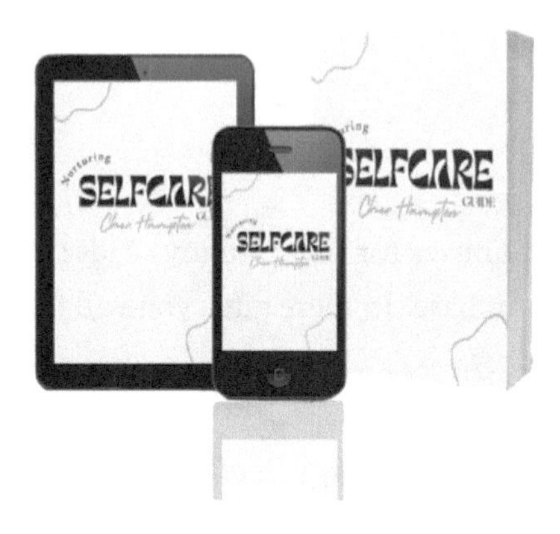

A Workbook with Special Meditations, Yoga Poses, and My Secret Self-Care Lists.

#3 Personality Development E-Course

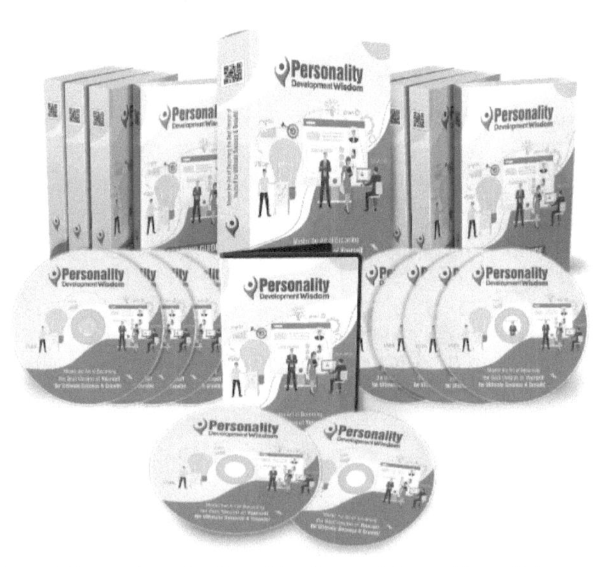

Master the Art of Becoming the Best Version of Yourself for Ultimate Success and Growth!

To receive this **bonus,** go to: https://booksforbetterlife.com/somatic-therapy-toolbox

Or scan the QR code:

Thank you!

I really appreciate you for purchasing my book!

You had the chance to pick a lot of other books, but you chose this one.

So, **thank you so much** for purchasing this book and reading it to the very last page! I hope that I was able to help you in your healing process, as my goal is to help as many people as possible!

Before you close the book, I want to ask for **a small favor**. Would you please consider ***leaving an honest review*** of the book? **This would be really helpful for me**, as I'm an independent author, and posting reviews is the best and easiest way to support me.

The feedback you provide will help me, and other readers, so I can continue selling, improving, and writing books. **It will mean the world to me to hear from you!**

Go to my book and scroll down (https://mybook.to/somatic-toolbox), or scan the QR code on the next page to leave a review:

Amazon US <—— ——> Amazon UK

Amazon CA <—— ——> Other Countries

References

Art therapy . (n.d.). Psychology Today. https://www.psychologytoday.com/za/therapy-types/art-therapy

Badendoch, B. (n.d.). *Somatic quotes*. Goodreads. https://www.goodreads.com/quotes/tag/somatic#:~:text=Life%20is%20always%20better%20in

Burnett-Zeigler, I., Schuette, S., Victorson, D., & Wisner, K. L. (2016). Mind–Body approaches to treating mental health symptoms among disadvantaged populations: A comprehensive review. *Journal of Alternative and Complementary Medicine, 22*(2), 115–124. https://doi.org/10.1089/acm.2015.0038

Grand, L. (n.d.). *Somatic quotes* . Goodreads. Retrieved March 10, 2024, from https://www.goodreads.com/quotes/tag/somatic#:~:text=Life%20is%20always%20better%20in

Greene, N. (2022, May 9). *Neuroplasticity and childhood trauma: Effects, healing, and EMDR*. Psych Central. https://psychcentral.com/ptsd/the-roles-neuroplasticity-and-emdr-play-in-healing-from-childhood-trauma

Johnson, G. (n.d.). *Somatic quotes*. Goodreads. https://www.goodreads.com/quotes/tag/somatic#:~:text=Life%20is%20always%20better%20in

Kristen Van Bael, Ball, M., Scarfo, J., & Emra Suleyman. (2023). Assessment of the mind-body connection: preliminary psychometric evidence for a new self-report questionnaire. *BMC Psychology, 11*(1). https://doi.org/10.1186/s4

0359-023-01302-3

Lynning, M., Svane, C., Westergaard, K., Bergien, S. O., Gunnersen, S. R., & Skovgaard, L. (2021). Tension and trauma releasing exercises for people with multiple sclerosis – An exploratory pilot study. *Journal of Traditional and Complementary Medicine, 11*(5), 383–389. https://doi.org/10.1016/j.jtcm e.2021.02.003

Maraboli, S. (2013). *Resilience quotes*. Goodreads. https://www.goodreads.co m/quotes/tag/resilience

Mehling, W. E., Wrubel, J., Daubenmier, J. J., Price, C. J., Kerr, C. E., Silow, T., Gopisetty, V., & Stewart, A. L. (2011). Body Awareness: a phenomenological inquiry into the common ground of mind-body therapies. *Philosophy, Ethics, and Humanities in Medicine, 6*(1), 6. https://doi.org/10.1186/1747-5341-6-6

Murakami, H. (2013). *Norwegian wood.* Random House Uk. (Original work published 1987)

Robinson, R. (n.d.). *Somatic quotes*. Goodreads. https://www.goodreads.com/ quotes/tag/somatic#:~:text=Life%20is%20always%20better%20in

Toussaint, L., Nguyen, Q. A., Roettger, C., Dixon, K., Offenbächer, M., Kohls, N., Hirsch, J., & Sirois, F. (2021). Effectiveness of progressive muscle relaxation, deep breathing, and guided imagery in promoting psychological and physiological states of relaxation. *Evidence-Based Complementary and Alternative Medicine, 2021*(1), 1–8. https://doi.org/10.1155/2021/5924040

Also by Cher Hampton

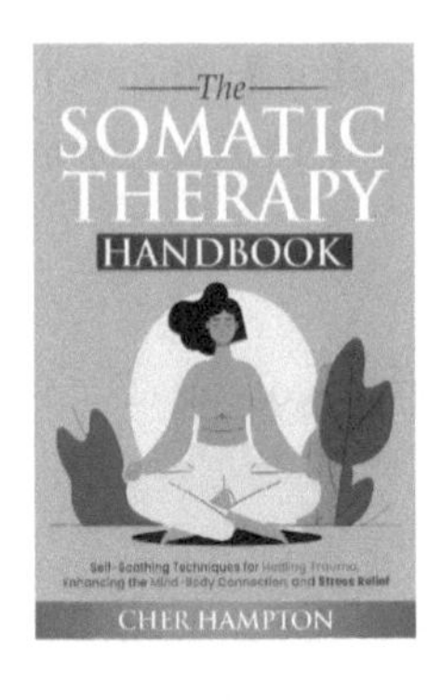

The Somatic Therapy Handbook

Discover the power of somatic therapy in this book. Dive into a transformative journey of healing trauma, nurturing the mind-body connection, and feeling more at ease in stressful times. **This comprehensive guide offers practical self-soothing techniques that empower you to navigate life's challenges with resilience and balance.**

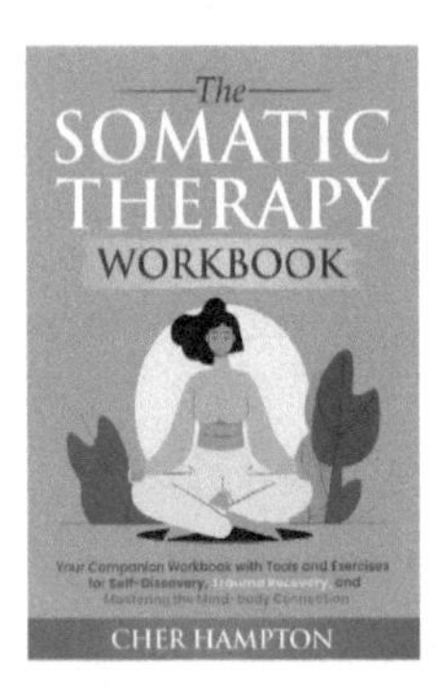

The Somatic Therapy Workbook

Why choose this workbook:

1) Comprehensive Companion: Perfectly complements *'The Somatic Therapy Handbook.'*

2) Practical Exercises: Hands-on tools for immediate impact.

3) Trauma-Informed: Gentle guidance for trauma recovery.

4) Mind-Body Mastery: Unleash the potential of the mind-body connection.

Made in United States
Troutdale, OR
06/29/2024